ABC OF COPD

ABC OF COPD

Edited by

GRAEME P CURRIE
Specialist registrar, Respiratory Unit, Aberdeen Royal Infirmary, Aberdeen

This book has been supplied by Boehringer Ingelheim and Pfizer as a service to continuing professional education.

The opinions expressed are those of the authors and do not necessarily reflect those of Boehringer Ingelheim and Pfizer.

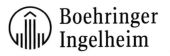

First published 2007

2   2007

Library of Congress Cataloging-in-Publication Data
ABC of COPD/edited by Graeme P. Currie.
        p. ; cm.
    Includes bibliographical references and index.
    ISBN 978-1-4051-4711-8 (alk. paper)
 1. Lungs–Diseases, Obstructive. I. Currie, Graeme P
    [DNLM: 1. Pulmonary Disease, Chronic Obstructive. WF 600 A134 2007]

  RC776.O3A23 2007
  616.2′4—dc22

                                            2006022493

ISBN 978-1-4051-4711-8

A catalogue record for this title is available from the British Library

Set by BMJ Electronic Production
Printed and bound in Spain by GraphyCems

Commissioning Editor: Mary Banks
Editorial Assistant: Vicky Pittman
Development Editor: Sally Carter/Charlie Hamlyn
Production Controller: Debbie Wyer
Senior technical editor: Greg Cotton

For further information on Blackwell Publishing, visit our website:
http://www.blackwellpublishing.com

Contents

Contributors

Peter J Barnes
Professor of respiratory medicine
National Heart and Lung Institute,
Imperial College, London

John Britton
Professor of epidemiology, University of Nottingham,
City Hospital, Nottingham

Gordon Christie
Consultant, Respiratory Unit,
Aberdeen Royal Infirmary, Aberdeen

Graeme P Currie
Specialist registrar, Respiratory Unit,
Aberdeen Royal Infirmary, Aberdeen

Graham Devereux
Senior lecturer and honorary consultant,
Department of Environmental and Occupational Medicine,
University of Aberdeen, Aberdeen

J Graham Douglas
Consultant, Respiratory Unit,
Aberdeen Royal Infirmary, Aberdeen

Daryl Freeman
Clinical Research Fellow,
Department of General Practice and Primary Care,
University of Aberdeen, Foresterhill Health Centre,
Aberdeen

Daniel K C Lee
Specialist Registrar,
Department of Respiratory Medicine,
Papworth Hospital, Papworth Everard,
Cambridge

Joe S Legge
Consultant, Respiratory Unit,
Aberdeen Royal Infirmary,
Aberdeen

Brian J Lipworth
Professor, Asthma and Allergy Research Group,
Division of Medicine and Therapeutics,
Ninewells Hospital and Medical School, Dundee

William MacNee
Professor of respiratory and
environmental medicine,
ELEGI, Colt Research,
MRC Centre for Inflammation Research,
Queen's Medical Research Institute,
University of Edinburgh, Edinburgh

Paul Plant
Consultant, Department of
respiratory medicine,
St James University Hospital, Leeds

David Price
Professor, Department of General Practice
and Primary Care, University of Aberdeen,
Foresterhill Health Centre, Aberdeen

Prasima Srivastava
Consultant, Respiratory Unit,
Aberdeen Royal Infirmary, Aberdeen

Jadwiga A Wedzicha
Professor, Academic Unit of Respiratory Medicine,
Royal Free and University College
Medical School, University College London,
London

Foreword

Chronic obstructive pulmonary disease (COPD) is a major global health problem. It already is the fourth commonest cause of death in industrialised countries and is soon predicted to become the third commonest cause of death worldwide. In the United Kingdom, the mortality from COPD in women now exceeds that of breast cancer. COPD is also predicted to become the fifth commonest cause of chronic disability, largely due to the increasing levels of cigarette smoking in developing countries in conjunction with an ageing population. It now affects about 6% of men and 4% of women in the United Kingdom and is one of the commonest causes of hospital admission. Because of this, COPD has an increasing economic impact, and its healthcare costs now exceed those of asthma by more than threefold. Despite these startling statistics, COPD has been relatively neglected and is still underdiagnosed in primary care settings. This is in marked contrast to asthma, which is now recognised and well managed in the community.

Highly effective treatment is available for asthma, which has in turn transformed patients' lives. Sadly this is not the case in COPD, where management is less effective and no drug has so far been shown to slow the relentless progression of the disease. However, important advances have been made in understanding the underlying disease process and in managing patients more effectively. In this volume of the ABC series, Graeme Currie and colleagues provide a timely update on the pathophysiology, diagnosis, and modern management of COPD. Once the disease has been diagnosed, a variety of non-pharmacological and pharmacological strategies can be implemented to try and improve the quality of life of patients. It is vital that COPD is recognised and treated appropriately in general practice where the majority of patients are managed, and this book provides a straightforward overview of the key issues relating to this important condition.

Peter J Barnes
Professor of Respiratory Medicine
National Heart and Lung Institute,
Imperial College, London

1 Definition, epidemiology, and risk factors

Graham Devereux

Definition

In 2004, the UK National Institute for Clinical Excellence defined chronic obstructive pulmonary disease (COPD) as "characterised by airflow obstruction. The airflow obstruction is usually progressive, not fully reversible and does not change markedly over several months. The disease is predominantly caused by smoking." COPD is the preferred umbrella term for the airflow obstruction associated with the diseases of chronic bronchitis and emphysema. These are closely related to, but not synonymous with, COPD.

Although asthma is associated with airflow obstruction, it is usually considered as a separate clinical entity. Some patients with chronic asthma also develop airflow obstruction that is relatively fixed (a consequence of airway remodelling) and often indistinguishable from COPD. Because of the high prevalence of asthma and COPD, they may coexist in many patients, creating diagnostic uncertainty. Other disease processes also associated with poorly reversible airflow obstruction include cystic fibrosis, bronchiectasis, and obliterative bronchiolitis. Although these conditions need to be considered in the differential diagnosis of obstructive airways disease, they are not conventionally covered by the definition of COPD.

Epidemiology

Prevalence

Estimating and comparing the prevalence of COPD in different countries is complicated by differences in its precise definition and in the level of underdiagnosis. For example, in the United Kingdom mild COPD is defined as the ratio of forced expiratory volume in 1 second (FEV_1) to the forced vital capacity (FVC) being <0.7 and the FEV_1 being 50-80% of the expected value. Other guidelines suggest slightly different spirometric values (see third article in this series).

A national UK study reported an abnormally low FEV_1 in 10% of men and 11% of women aged 16-65 years. Similarly, a study in Manchester found non-reversible airflow obstruction in 11% of adults aged >45, of whom 65% had not had COPD diagnosed. In the United States the reported prevalence of airflow obstruction with an FEV_1 $<80\%$ of the expected value is 6.8%, with 1.5% of the population having an FEV_1 $<50\%$ of expected and 0.5% having more severe obstruction (FEV_1 $<35\%$ of expected). As in the UK, about 60% of those with airflow obstruction had not had COPD diagnosed. As much as 40-50% of the actual prevalence of COPD, based on measurements of ventilatory function, may be undiagnosed; many people present relatively late with moderate or severe airflow obstruction.

In England and Wales some 900 000 people have COPD diagnosed—so, after allowing for underdiagnosis, the true number is likely to be about 1.5 million. The mean age at diagnosis in the UK is roughly 67 years, and prevalence increases with age. COPD is more common in men than women and is associated with socioeconomic deprivation. The prevalence of diagnosed COPD in women is increasing (from 0.8% in 1990 to 1.4% in 1997), whereas in men it seems to have reached a plateau since the middle 1990s. Similar trends have been reported in the US. These trends in prevalence probably reflect sex differences in cigarette smoking since the 1970s.

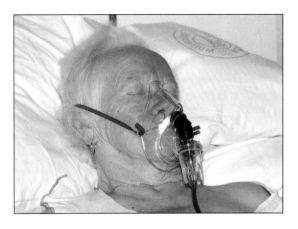

Definitions of conditions associated with airflow obstruction

Chronic obstructive pulmonary disease (COPD)—Airflow obstruction that is usually progressive, not reversible, and does not change markedly over several months. It is predominantly caused by smoking

Chronic bronchitis—Presence of chronic productive cough on most days for 3 months, in each of 2 consecutive years, and other causes of productive cough have been excluded

Emphysema—Abnormal, permanent enlargement of the distal airspaces, distal to the terminal bronchioles, accompanied by destruction of their walls and without obvious fibrosis

Asthma—Widespread narrowing of the bronchial airways which changes its severity over short periods either spontaneously or after treatment

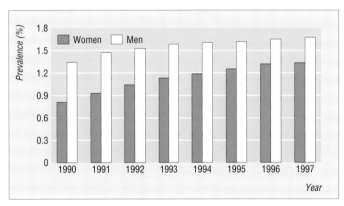

Prevalence of diagnosed COPD in UK men and women during 1990-7

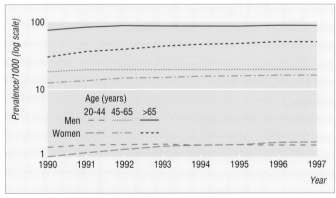

Prevalence of diagnosed COPD in UK men and women by age, during 1990-7

ABC of chronic obstructive pulmonary disease

Mortality

COPD is the fourth leading cause of death in the US and Europe. With the increase in cigarette smoking in developing countries, especially China, it is expected to become the third leading cause of death worldwide by 2020. During 2003, about 26 000 people died from COPD in the UK, accounting for 4.9% of all deaths, with 14 000 of these deaths occurring in men and 12 000 in women. These represent 5.4% of all male deaths and 4.2% of all female deaths.

In the UK over the past 30 years, mortality has fallen in men and risen in women, although the sex difference will probably disappear in the near future. In the US, mortality in women has also risen substantially, from 20.1 to 56.7 per 100 000 between 1980 and 2000, while in men the increase has been more modest, from 73.0 to 82.6 per 100 000. In 2000, for the first time, more women than men died from COPD (59 936 v 59 118). Mortality increases with age, disease severity, and socioeconomic disadvantage. On average, COPD reduces life expectancy by 1.8 years in the UK (76.5 v 78.3 years for controls)—mild disease reducing it by 1.1 years, moderate disease by 1.7 years, and severe disease by 4.1 years.

Morbidity and economic impact

The morbidity and economic costs associated with COPD are high, largely unrecognised, and more than twice those from asthma. The impact on quality of life is particularly high in patients with frequent exacerbations, and even patients with mild disease have an impaired quality of life.

Since the mid-1990s, emergency admissions have increased by at least 50%, so that in 2002-3 there were 110 000 hospital admissions for an exacerbation of COPD in England, accounting for 1.1 million bed days. At least 10% of emergency admissions to hospital are as a consequence of COPD, and this proportion is even greater during the winter. Most admissions are of people older than 65 years with advanced disease, who are often admitted repeatedly and use a disproportionate amount of resources. About 25% of patients with COPD diagnosed need admission to hospital, with some 15% of patients being admitted each year.

The impact in primary care is even greater, with 86% of care being provided exclusively by primary care. An average general practitioner's list will contain some 200 patients (even more in areas of social deprivation), although not all will have it diagnosed. On average, patients make six or seven visits annually to their general practitioner. Each patient costs the UK economy an estimated £1639 annually, equating to a national burden of £982m (€1450, $1741m). For each patient, annual direct costs to the NHS are £819, with 54% of this being due to hospital admissions and 19% due to drug treatment. COPD results in further costs to society in that roughly 40% of UK patients are below retirement age, and the disease prevents about 25% from working and reduces the capacity to work in a further 10%. Annual indirect costs have been estimated at £820 per patient and consist of the cost of disability, absence from work, premature mortality, and the time caregivers miss work.

Risk factors

Smoking

Cigarette smoking is clearly the single most important risk factor in the development of COPD. Current smoking is also associated with an increased risk of death. Pipe and cigar smoking also significantly increase morbidity and mortality from COPD, though the risk is less than for cigarettes. Around half of cigarette smokers develop some airflow obstruction, despite the fact that only 10-20% develop clinically significant

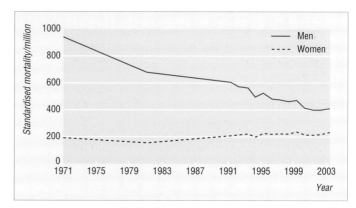

UK mortality from COPD since 1971

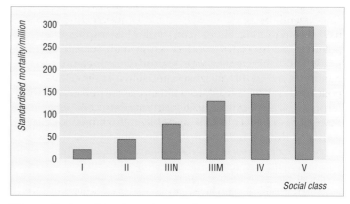

UK mortality from COPD by socioeconomic status

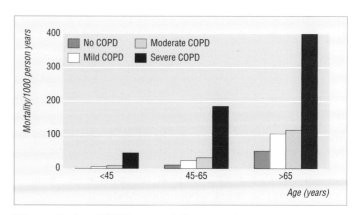

UK mortality from COPD by age and disease severity

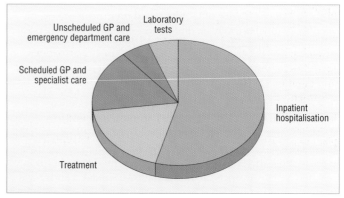

Direct costs of COPD to the NHS

COPD. Although smoking is the most important risk factor, it is not a prerequisite: COPD can occur in non-smokers with longstanding asthma or with α_1 antitrypsin deficiency. Moreover, about 20% of cases in men are not attributable to smoking.

A more contentious issue is the possible relation between environmental tobacco smoke and development of COPD: several case-control studies have shown a trend towards an increased risk of COPD with passive smoking. However, the adverse effect of maternal smoking on childhood ventilatory function is clearer: smoking during and after pregnancy is associated with reduced infant, childhood, and adult ventilatory function. Most studies have shown that the effects of antenatal smoking are greater in magnitude than, and independent of, the effects of postnatal exposure.

Air pollution

Urban air pollution may affect lung function development and consequently be a risk factor for COPD. Cross sectional studies have shown that higher concentrations of atmospheric air pollution are associated with increased cough, sputum production, and breathlessness and reduced ventilatory function. Exposure to particulate and nitrogen dioxide air pollution has been associated with impaired ventilatory function in adults and reduced lung growth in children. In developing countries indoor air pollution from biomass fuel (used for cooking and heating) has been implicated as a risk factor for COPD, particularly in women.

Occupation

Intense prolonged exposure to dusts and chemicals can cause COPD independently of cigarette smoking, though smoking seems to enhance the effects of such occupational exposure. About 20% of diagnosed cases of COPD are thought to be attributable to occupation; in lifelong non-smokers this proportion increases to 30%. Exposure to noxious gases and particles—such as grain, isocyanates, cadmium, coal, other mineral dusts, and welding fumes—have been implicated in the development of chronic airflow obstruction. Thus, a full chronological occupational history should be taken, as relevant occupational exposures are often missed by clinicians.

α_1 antitrypsin deficiency

The best documented genetic risk factor for COPD is α_1 antitrypsin deficiency. However, this is rare and is present in only 1-2% of patients. α_1 antitrypsin is a glycoprotein responsible for most of the antiprotease activity in serum. Its gene is highly polymorphic, but some genotypes (usually ZZ) are associated with low serum concentrations (typically 10-20% of normal). Severe deficiency of α_1 antitrypsin is associated with premature and accelerated development of COPD in smokers and non-smokers, though the rate of decline in lung function is greatly accelerated in those who smoke.

The α_1 antitrypsin status of patients with severe COPD who are less than 40 years old should be determined since over half of such patients have this deficiency. Detection of such cases identifies family members who will require genetic counselling and patients who might be suitable for future potential treatment with α_1 antitrypsin replacement.

Competing interests: GPC has received funding for attending international conferences and honoraria for giving talks from pharmaceutical companies GlaxoSmithKline, Pfizer, and AstraZeneca.

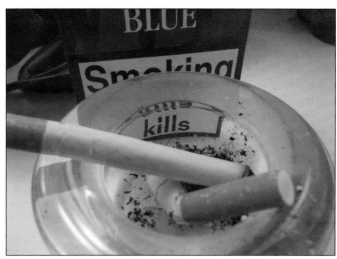

Current cigarette smoking is the most important risk factor for the development of COPD

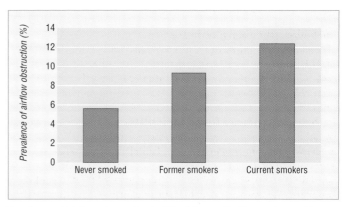

Prevalence of airflow obstruction in US adults aged >17 years by smoking status

Further reading

- Anto JM, Vermiere P, Vestbo J, Sunyer J. Epidemiology of chronic obstructive pulmonary disease. *Eur Respir J* 2001;17:982-94
- Britton M. The burden of COPD in the UK: results from the confronting COPD survey. *Respir Med* 2003;97(suppl C):S71-9
- Pride NB, Soriano JB. Chronic obstructive pulmonary disease in the United Kingdom: trends in mortality, morbidity and smoking. *Curr Opin Pulm Med* 2002;8:95-101
- National Collaborating Centre for Chronic Conditions. National clinical guideline on management of chronic obstructive pulmonary disease in adults in primary and secondary care. *Thorax* 2004;59(suppl 1):1-3, 192-4
- Chapman RS, He X, Blair AE, Lan Q. Improvement in household stoves and risk of chronic obstructive pulmonary disease in Xuanwei, China: retrospective cohort study. *BMJ* 2005;331:1050-2.

The figure of a COPD patient wearing a facemask was supplied by Mediscan. The figures of prevalence of COPD in UK men and women and of deaths from COPD by age and disease severity are adapted from Soriano JB, et al, *Thorax* 2000; 55:789-94. The data for the figures of UK mortality from COPD and of mortality from COPD by socioeconomic status are from *Mortality statistics: cause. Review by the registrar general on deaths by cause, sex and age, in England and Wales, 2003.* London: Office for National Statistics, 2004. The data for the diagram of management costs of COPD are from Britton M, *Resp Med* 2003;97(suppl C): S71-9. The data for the figure of prevalence of airflow obstruction by smoking status are from Mannino DM, et al, *Arch Intern Med* 2000;1601683-9.

2 Pathology, pathogenesis, and pathophysiology

William MacNee

Pathology

Chronic obstructive pulmonary disease (COPD) is characterised by poorly reversible airflow obstruction and an abnormal inflammatory response in the lungs. The latter represents the innate and adaptive immune responses to long term exposure to noxious particles and gases, particularly cigarette smoke. All cigarette smokers have some inflammation in their lungs, but those who develop COPD have an enhanced or abnormal response to inhaling toxic agents. This amplified response may result in mucous hypersecretion (chronic bronchitis), tissue destruction (emphysema), and disruption of normal repair and defence mechanisms causing small airway inflammation and fibrosis (bronchiolitis).

These pathological changes result in increased resistance to airflow in the small conducting airways, increased compliance of the lungs, air trapping, and progressive airflow obstruction—all characteristic features of COPD. We have good understanding of the cellular and molecular mechanisms underlying the pathological changes found in COPD.

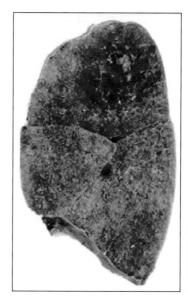

Sagital slice of lung removed from a patient who received a lung transplant for COPD. Centrilobular lesions have coalesced to produce severe lung destruction in the upper lobe

---

Pathological changes found in COPD

Proximal cartilaginous airways (>2 mm in diameter)
- Increased numbers of macrophages and CD8 T lymphocytes
- Few neutrophils and eosinophils (neutrophils increase with progressive disease)
- Submucosal bronchial gland enlargement and goblet cell metaplasia (results in excessive mucous production or chronic bronchitis)
- Cellular infiltrates (neutrophils and lymphocytes) of bronchial glands
- Airway epithelial squamous metaplasia, ciliary dysfunction, hypertrophy of smooth muscle and connective tissue

Peripheral airways (non-cartilaginous airways <2 mm diameter)
- Increased numbers of macrophages and T lymphocytes (CD8 > CD4)
- Increased numbers of B lymphocytes, lymphoid follicles, and fibroblasts
- Few neutrophils or eosinophils
- Bronchiolitis at an early stage
- Luminal and inflammatory exudates
- Pathological extension of goblet cells and squamous metaplasia into peripheral airways
- Peribronchial fibrosis and airway narrowing with progressive disease

Lung parenchyma (respiratory bronchioles and alveoli)
- Increased numbers of macrophages and CD8 T lymphocytes
- Alveolar wall destruction from loss of epithelial and endothelial cells
- Development of emphysema (abnormal enlargement of airspaces distal to terminal bronchioles)
- Microscopic emphysematous changes:
  Centrilobular—dilatation and destruction of respiratory bronchioles (commonly found in smokers and predominantly in upper zones)
  Panacinar—destruction of the whole acinus (commonly found in α_1 antitrypsin deficiency and more common in lower zones)
- Macroscopic emphysematous changes:
  Microscopic changes progress to bulla formation (defined as an emphysematous airspace > 1 cm in diameter)

Pulmonary vasculature
- Increased numbers of macrophages and T lymphocytes
- Early changes—Intimal thickening, endothelial dysfunction
- Late changes—Hypertrophy of vascular smooth muscle, collagen deposition, destruction of capillary bed, development of pulmonary hypertension and cor pulmonale

---

Pathogenesis

Inflammation is present in the lungs, particularly the small airways, of all people who smoke. This normal protective response to the inhaled toxins is amplified in COPD, leading to tissue destruction, impairment of the defence mechanisms that limit such destruction, and disruption of the repair mechanisms. In general, the inflammatory and structural changes in the airways increase with disease severity and persist even after smoking cessation. Besides inflammation, two other processes are involved in the pathogenesis of COPD—an imbalance between proteases and antiproteases and an imbalance between oxidants and antioxidants (oxidative stress) in the lungs.

Inflammatory cells

COPD is characterised by increased numbers of neutrophils, macrophages, and T lymphocytes (CD8 more than CD4) in the

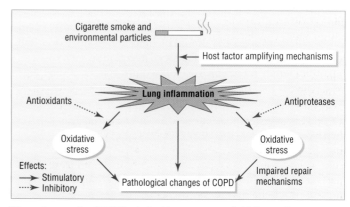

The pathogenesis of COPD; dashed bars represent inhibitory effects

lungs. In general, the extent of the inflammation is related to the degree of the airflow obstruction. These inflammatory cells release a variety of cytokines and mediators that participate in the disease process. This inflammatory pattern is markedly different from that seen in patients with asthma.

Inflammatory mediators
Many inflammatory mediators are increased in COPD, including
- Leucotriene B₄, a neutrophil and T cell chemoattractant which is produced by macrophages, neutrophils, and epithelial cells
- Chemotactic factors such as the CXC chemokines interleukin 8 and growth related oncogene α, which are produced by macrophages and epithelial cells. These attract cells from the circulation and amplify pro-inflammatory responses
- Pro-inflammatory cytokines such as tumour necrosis factor α and interleukins 1β and 6
- Growth factors such as transforming growth factor β, which may cause fibrosis in the airways either directly or through release of another cytokine, connective tissue growth factor.

Protease and antiprotease imbalance
Increased production (or activity) of proteases and inactivation (or reduced production) of antiproteases results in imbalance. Cigarette smoke, and inflammation itself, produce oxidative stress, which primes several inflammatory cells to release a combination of proteases and inactivates several antiproteases by oxidation. The main proteases involved are those produced by neutrophils (including the serine proteases elastase, cathepsin G, and protease 3) and macrophages (cysteine proteases and cathepsins E, A, L, and S), and various matrix metalloproteases (MMP-8, MMP-9, and MMP-12). The main antiproteases involved in the pathogenesis of emphysema include α₁ antitrypsin, secretory leucoprotease inhibitor, and tissue inhibitors of metalloproteases.

Oxidative stress
The oxidative burden is increased in COPD. Sources of oxidants include cigarette smoke and reactive oxygen and nitrogen species released from inflammatory cells. This creates an imbalance in oxidants and antioxidants of oxidative stress. Many markers of oxidative stress are increased in stable COPD and are further increased in exacerbations. Oxidative stress can lead to inactivation of antiproteases or stimulation of mucous production. It can also amplify inflammation by enhancing transcription factor activation (such as nuclear factor κB) and hence gene expression of pro-inflammatory mediators.

Pathophysiology
The above pathogenic mechanisms result in the pathological changes found in COPD. These in turn result in physiological abnormalities—mucous hypersecretion and ciliary dysfunction, airflow obstruction and hyperinflation, gas exchange abnormalities, pulmonary hypertension, and systemic effects.

Mucous hypersecretion and ciliary dysfunction
Mucous hypersecretion results in a chronic productive cough. This is characteristic of chronic bronchitis but not necessarily associated with airflow obstruction, and not all patients with COPD have symptomatic mucous hypersecretion. The hypersecretion is due to squamous metaplasia, increased numbers of goblet cells, and increased size of bronchial submucosal glands in response to chronic irritation by noxious particles and gases. Ciliary dysfunction is due to squamous metaplasia of epithelial cells and results in an abnormal mucociliary escalator and difficulty in expectorating.

Inflammatory cells and mediators in COPD
- Neutrophils, which release proteases, are increased in the sputum and distal airspaces of smokers; a further increase occurs in COPD and is related to disease severity
- Macrophages, which produce inflammatory mediators and proteases, are increased in number in airways, lung parenchyma, and in bronchoalveolar lavage fluid
- T lymphocytes (CD4 and CD8 cells) are increased in the airways and lung parenchyma, with an increase in CD8:CD4 ratio. Numbers of Th1 and Tc1 cells, which produce interferon γ, also increase. CD8 cells may be cytotoxic and cause alveolar wall destruction
- B lymphocytes are increased in the peripheral airways and within lymphoid follicles, possibly as a response to chronic infection of the airways.

Proteases and antiproteases involved in COPD

Proteases	Antiproteases
Serine proteases	α₁ antitrypsin
Neutrophil elastase	
Cathepsin G	Secretory leucoprotease inhibitor
Protease 3	Elafin
Cysteine proteases	Cystatins
Cathepsins B, K, L, S	
Matrix metalloproteases (MMP-8, MMP-9, MMP-12)	Tissue inhibitors of MMP (TIMP1-4)

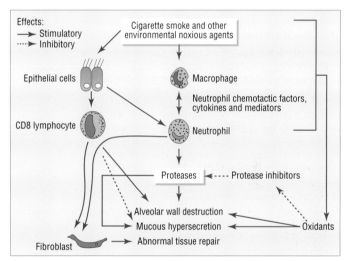

Inflammatory mechanisms in COPD. Cigarette smoke activates macrophages and epithelial cells to release chemotactic factors that recruit neutrophils and CD8 cells from the circulation. These cells release factors that activate fibroblasts, resulting in abnormal repair processes and bronchiolar fibrosis. An imbalance between proteases released from neutrophils and macrophages and antiproteases leads to alveolar wall destruction (emphysema). Proteases also cause the release of mucous. An increased oxidant burden, resulting from smoke inhalation or release of oxidants from inflammatory leucocytes, causes epithelial and other cells to release chemotactic factors, inactivate antiproteases, and directly injure alveolar walls and cause mucous secretion

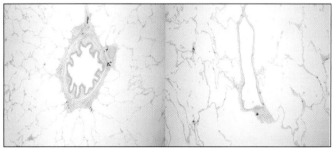

Left: Normal small airway with alveolar attachments. Right: Emphysematous airway, with loss of alveolar walls, enlargement of alveolar spaces, and decreased alveolar wall attachment

ABC of chronic obstructive pulmonary disease

Airflow obstruction and hyperinflation or air trapping

The main site of airflow obstruction occurs in the small conducting airways that are <2 mm in diameter. This is because of inflammation and narrowing (airway remodelling) and inflammatory exudates in the small airways. Other factors contributing to airflow obstruction include loss of the lung elastic recoil (due to destruction of alveolar walls) and destruction of alveolar support (from alveolar attachments).

The airway obstruction progressively traps air during expiration, resulting in hyperinflation at rest and dynamic hyperinflation during exercise. Hyperinflation reduces the inspiratory capacity and therefore the functional residual capacity during exercise. These features result in breathlessness and limited exercise capacity typical of COPD. The airflow obstruction in COPD is best measured by spirometry and is a prerequisite for its diagnosis.

Gas exchange abnormalities

These occur in advanced disease and are characterised by arterial hypoxaemia with or without hypercapnia. An abnormal distribution of ventilation:perfusion ratios—due to the anatomical changes found in COPD—is the main mechanism for abnormal gas exchange. The extent of impairment of diffusing capacity for carbon monoxide per litre of alveolar volume correlates well with the severity of emphysema.

Pulmonary hypertension

This develops late in COPD, at the time of severe gas exchange abnormalities. Contributing factors include pulmonary arterial constriction (as a result of hypoxia), endothelial dysfunction, remodelling of the pulmonary arteries (smooth muscle hypertrophy and hyperplasia), and destruction of the pulmonary capillary bed. Structural changes in the pulmonary arterioles result in persistent pulmonary hypertension and right ventricular hypertrophy or enlargement and dysfunction (cor pulmonale).

Systemic effects of COPD

Systemic inflammation and skeletal muscle wasting contribute to limiting the exercise capacity of patients and worsen the prognosis irrespective of degree of airflow obstruction. Patients also have an increased risk of cardiovascular disease, which is associated with an increase in C reactive protein.

Pathophysiology of exacerbations

Exacerbations are often associated with increased neutrophilic inflammation and, in some mild exacerbations, increased numbers of eosinophils. Exacerbations can be caused by infection (bacterial or viral), air pollution, and changes in ambient temperature.

In mild exacerbations, airflow obstruction is unchanged or only slightly increased. Severe exacerbations are associated with worsening of pulmonary gas exchange due to increased inequality between ventilation and perfusion and subsequent respiratory muscle fatigue. The worsening ventilation-perfusion relation results from airway inflammation, oedema, mucous hypersecretion, and bronchoconstriction. These reduce ventilation and cause hypoxic vasoconstriction of pulmonary arterioles, which in turn impairs perfusion.

Respiratory muscle fatigue and alveolar hypoventilation can contribute to hypoxaemia, hypercapnia, and respiratory acidosis, and lead to severe respiratory failure and death. Hypoxia and respiratory acidosis can induce pulmonary vasoconstriction, which increases the load on the right ventricle and, together with renal and hormonal changes, results in peripheral oedema.

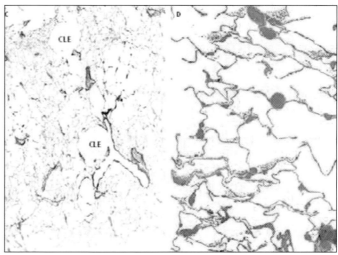

Left: Low power photomicrograph of the early changes of centrilobular emphysema (CLE) that have destroyed central portions of several acini of a single secondary lobule. Right: Slightly higher power photomicrograph showing the more even destruction of the lobule in panacinar emphysema

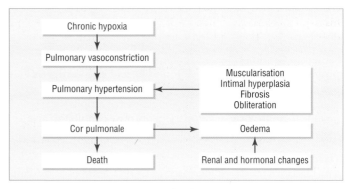

Development of pulmonary hypertension in COPD

Systemic features of COPD

- Cachexia
- Skeletal muscle wasting and disuse atrophy
- Increased risk of cardiovascular disease (associated with increased concentrations of C reactive protein)
- Normochromic normocytic anaemia
- Secondary polycythaemia
- Osteoporosis
- Depression and anxiety

Competing interests: GPC has received funding for attending international conferences and honoraria for giving talks from pharmaceutical companies GlaxoSmithKline, Pfizer, and AstraZeneca.

The pictures of a mid-saggital slice of lung removed from a patient with COPD and of the early changes of centrilobular emphysema and of panacinar emphysema are reproduced with permission from Hogg JC. *Lancet* 2004;364: 709-21. The pictures of normal small airway and of emphysematous airway are reproduced with permission from W MacNee and D Lamb.

3   Diagnosis

Graeme P Currie, Joe S Legge

As with most other common medical conditions, the diagnosis of chronic obstructive pulmonary disease (COPD) depends on a consistent history and appropriate examination findings. Confirmatory objective evidence is provided by spirometry. Doctors should consider the possibility of COPD in any patient aged 35 years or older with any relevant respiratory symptom and a history of smoking.

History

Consider COPD in any current or former smoker age >35 years who complains of any combination of breathlessness, chest tightness, wheeze, sputum production, cough, frequent chest infections, and impaired exercise tolerance.

COPD may also be present in the absence of noticeable symptoms, so look for it in individuals who are current or former smokers. Pay particular attention to features in the history or examination that may suggest an alternative or concomitant diagnosis. Since asthma tends to be the main condition in the differential diagnosis of COPD, a careful history should be taken in order to help distinguish between the disorders. Ask about previous and present occupations, particularly with regard to exposure to dusts and chemicals.

Record the patient's current smoking status and calculate the number of smoking pack years.
- Number of pack years = (number of cigarettes smoked/day × number of years smoked)/20
- For example: a patient who has smoked 15 cigarettes a day for 40 years has a $(15 \times 40)/20 = 30$ pack year smoking history.

Calculating the number of smoking pack years overcomes the problems of differences in duration and intensity of cigarette smoking. The decline in forced expiratory volume in 1 second (FEV_1) is generally related to the extent of cumulative exposure, although there is wide variability between individuals.

As part of the overall assessment of COPD, find out about symptoms of anxiety and depression, other medical conditions, current drug treatments, frequency of exacerbations, previous hospitalisations, exercise limitation, number of days missed from work and their financial impact, and extent of social and family support. COPD causes systemic effects, with weight loss being an under-recognised symptom in advanced disease.

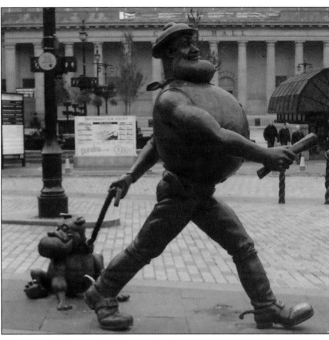

Patients with advanced COPD can develop an increased anteroposterior chest diameter—a barrel shaped chest

Differences between COPD and asthma

	COPD	Asthma
Age	>35 years	Any age
Cough	Persistent and productive	Intermittent and non-productive
Smoking	Almost invariable	Possible
Breathlessness	Progressive and persistent	Intermittent and variable
Nocturnal symptoms	Uncommon unless in severe disease	Common
Family history	Uncommon unless family members also smoke	Common
Concomitant eczema or allergic rhinitis	Possible	Common

Conditions in the differential diagnosis of COPD

Asthma
Suggestive features—Family history, atopy, non-smoker, young age, nocturnal symptoms
Investigation—Peak flow monitoring, reversibility testing

Congestive heart failure
Suggestive features—Orthopnoea, history of ischaemic heart disease, fine lung crackles
Investigation—Chest radiograph, electrocardiogram, echocardiogram

Lung cancer
Suggestive features—Haemoptysis, weight loss, hoarseness
Investigation—Chest radiograph, bronchoscopy, computed tomography

Bronchiectasis
Suggestive features—Copious sputum production, frequent chest infections, childhood pneumonia, coarse lung crackles
Investigation—Sputum microscopy, culture, and sensitivity; high resolution computed tomography

Interstitial lung disease
Suggestive features—Dry cough; history of connective tissue disease; use of drugs such as methotrexate, amiodarone, etc; fine lung crackles
Investigation—Pulmonary function testing, chest radiograph, high resolution computed tomography, lung biopsy, test for autoantibodies

Opportunistic infection
Suggestive features—Dry cough, risk factors for immunosuppression, fever
Investigation—Chest radiograph; sputum microscopy, culture, and sensitivity; induced sputum; bronchoalveolar lavage

Tuberculosis
Suggestive features—Weight loss, haemoptysis, night sweats, risk factors for tuberculosis and immunosuppression
Investigation—Chest radiograph; sputum microscopy, culture, and sensitivity

Examination

Because of the heterogeneity of COPD, patients may show a range of phenotypic clinical pictures. However, physical examination can be normal especially in patients with mild disease, although it may help suggest an alternative or coexistent diagnosis. Moreover, features of advanced airflow obstruction—peripheral and central cyanosis, hyperinflated chest, pursed lip breathing, accessory muscle use, wheeze, diminished breath sounds, and paradoxical movement of the lower ribs—are found in other chronic respiratory conditions and are therefore of low diagnostic sensitivity and specificity.

Cor pulmonale is defined as right ventricular hypertrophy due to any chronic lung disorder. Some patients with severe COPD may show signs consistent with cor pulmonale (raised jugular venous pressure, loud P_2 heart sounds due to pulmonary hypertension, tricuspid regurgitation, pitting peripheral oedema, and hepatomegaly). Look for skeletal muscle wasting and cachexia, which may be present in those with advanced disease. Finger clubbing is not found in COPD, and its presence should prompt thorough evaluation to exclude a cause such as lung cancer, bronchiectasis, or idiopathic pulmonary fibrosis. At presentation, record the weight and height and calculate the body mass index (weight (kg)/(height (m)^2)). It is categorised for both men and women as < 18.5 for underweight, 18.5-24.9 for normal, 25-29.9 for overweight, and ≥ 30 for obese.

Investigations

Peak expiratory flow
Solitary peak expiratory flow readings can seriously underestimate the extent of airflow obstruction, while serial monitoring of peak expiratory flow is not generally useful in the diagnosis of COPD.

Spirometry
While history and examination are necessary in the diagnostic work up, showing airflow obstruction is vital in confirming the diagnosis. Spirometry should be arranged in all patients with suspected COPD. It is increasingly performed in primary care and can be carried out with minimal training for both clinician and patient. It measures
- Forced vital capacity (FVC)—the maximum volume of air forcibly exhaled after full inspiration (that is, from total lung capacity)
- Forced expiratory volume in one second (FEV_1)—the volume of air exhaled during the first second of the FVC manoeuvre
- The FEV_1/FVC ratio.

Compare the FEV_1 and FVC with predicted normal values for age, height, and sex. These measures are often expressed as the percentage predicted as well as in absolute values in litres. Airflow obstruction is present if the FEV_1/FVC ratio is < 0.7 and the FEV_1 is < 80% of the predicted value. A ratio of ≥ 0.7 is either normal or suggestive of a restrictive ventilatory defect.

Spirometry also allows patients with COPD to be categorised according to severity, and enables monitoring of changes in lung function over time and the response to treatment. If spirometric values return to normal after treatment then clinically significant COPD is not present.

Reversibility testing
Patients with COPD used to be categorised by their response to a therapeutic trial of corticosteroids. However, it is now known that an improvement in lung function after a short course of oral corticosteroids usually fails to predict future benefit from

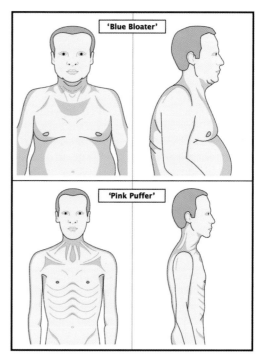

The clinical heterogeneity of COPD: a typical "blue bloater" (top) and "pink puffer" (bottom)

Common causes of obstructive and restrictive spirometry

Obstructive disorders
- COPD
- Asthma
- Bronchiectasis

Restrictive disorders
- Neuromuscular disease
- Previous pneumonectomy
- Interstitial lung disease
- Pleural effusion
- Kyphoscoliosis
- Obesity

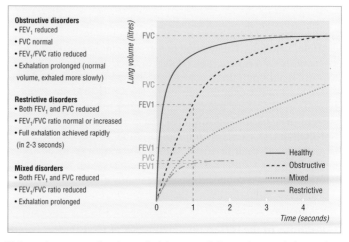

Volume time curves showing typical features of obstructive, restrictive, and mixed obstructive-restrictive ventilatory disorders

Categorisation of COPD severity by different guidelines

Airflow obstruction	% of predicted FEV_1*		
	BTS	ATS-ERS	GOLD
Mild	50-80%	≥ 80%	≥ 80%
Moderate	30-49%	50-80%	30-79%
Severe	< 30%	30-50%	< 30%
Very severe		< 30%	

*FEV_1/FVC ratio should be < 0.7 in all cases.
BTS = British Thoracic Society. ATS-ERS = American Thoracic Society and European Respiratory Society. GOLD = Global Initiative for Chronic Obstructive Lung Disease. The ATS/ERS guidelines also suggest an "at risk" group—smokers with typical symptoms of COPD with an FEV_1/FVC ratio > 0.7 and FEV_1 ≥ 80% predicted. The GOLD guidelines suggest an "at risk" category in smokers with typical symptoms of COPD but normal spirometry

long term inhaled corticosteroids. Reversibility testing to oral corticosteroids or inhaled bronchodilator is not always necessary, but it should be performed if asthma is thought likely or if the response to treatment (β_2 agonists or corticosteroids) is surprisingly good. However, asthma can often be distinguished from COPD by the history, examination, and baseline spirometry.

More detailed lung function measurements such as lung volumes (total lung capacity and residual volume), gas transfer coefficient, and walking distance in six minutes can be done if diagnostic doubt persists or more thorough evaluation is required.

Imaging

At the time of diagnosis, arrange a chest radiograph in all patients. This is useful in excluding other conditions as a cause of respiratory symptoms and may show typical features of COPD. When there is diagnostic doubt or a surgical procedure is contemplated (such as lung volume reduction surgery or bullectomy) computed tomography of the chest is required.

Other tests

A full blood count should be arranged. This may show secondary polycythaemia, which can result from chronic hypoxaemia, and it is important to exclude anaemia as a cause of breathlessness. A raised eosinophil count suggests the possibility of an alternative diagnosis such as asthma.

In patients with signs of cor pulmonale, electrocardiography may show typical changes of chronic right sided heart strain. However, echocardiography is more sensitive in detecting tricuspid valve incompetence, as well as right atrial and ventricular hypertrophy, and may indirectly assess pulmonary artery pressure. It is also useful in determining whether left ventricular dysfunction is present, especially when the spirometric impairment is disproportional to the extent of breathlessness. Ischaemic heart disease may be the sole or contributory cause of breathlessness even in the absence of chest pain, and investigations should be tailored accordingly. Indeed, dyspnoea due to causes other than COPD should be considered when the extent of physical limitation seems disproportionate to the degree of airflow obstruction, or in patients with normal oxygen saturation who have little or no fall in levels during a six minute walk.

Patients with a family history of COPD or in whom it presents at a young age (especially when smoking pack years are negligible) should have their α_1 antitrypsin concentrations measured. If α_1 antitrypsin deficiency is discovered, appropriate family screening and counselling is advised.

Pulse oximetry is useful in most patients, especially those with advanced disease (such as $FEV_1 < 50\%$ predicted) or polycythaemia, in order to check for significant hypoxaemia. Patients with a resting oxygen saturation of $< 92\%$ should have measurement of arterial blood gases and, where necessary and appropriate, be assessed for long term domiciliary or ambulatory oxygen therapy.

Competing interests: GPC has received funding for attending international conferences and honorariums for giving talks from pharmaceutical companies GlaxoSmithKline, Pfizer, and AstraZeneca.

Changes in lung function consistent with a diagnosis of asthma

- Improvement in FEV_1 by $\geq 15\%$ and ≥ 200 ml (or in peak expiratory flow of $\geq 20\%$ and ≥ 60 l/min) 20 minutes after taking 400 µg (2 puffs) inhaled salbutamol or 2.5 mg nebulised salbutamol
- Improvement in FEV_1 by $\geq 15\%$ and ≥ 200 ml (or in peak expiratory flow of $\geq 20\%$ and ≥ 60 l/min) after taking 30 mg oral prednisolone for two weeks
- Variability in peak expiratory flow (difference between highest and lowest scores) of $\geq 20\%$ during three consecutive days over two weeks

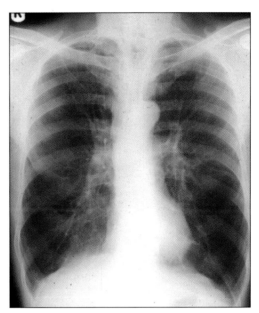

Chest radiograph showing typical changes of COPD (hyperinflated lung fields, flat diaphragms, prominent pulmonary arteries, increased translucency of lung fields and "squared off" lung apices)

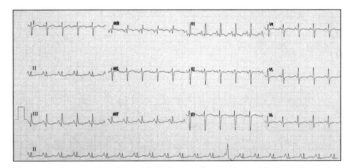

Electrocardiogram showing typical changes in a patient with cor pulmonale secondary to advanced COPD (p-pulmonale, right axis deviation, partial right bundle branch block, dominant R wave in lead V1)

Further reading

- National clinical guideline on management of chronic obstructive pulmonary disease in adults in primary and secondary care. *Thorax* 2004;59(suppl 1):1-232.
- Celli BR, MacNee W. Standards for the diagnosis and treatment of patients with COPD: a summary of the ATS/ERS position paper. *Eur Respir J* 2004;23:932-46.
- Pauwels RA, Buist AS, Calverley PM, Jenkins CR, Hurd SS. Global strategy for the diagnosis, management, and prevention of chronic obstructive pulmonary disease. NHLBI/WHO Global Initiative for Chronic Obstructive Lung Disease (GOLD) Workshop summary. *Am J Respir Crit Care Med* 2001;163:1256-76.
- British guideline on the management of asthma. *Thorax* 2003;58 (suppl 1):i1-94.
- Pauwels RA, Rabe KF. Burden and clinical features of chronic obstructive pulmonary disease (COPD). *Lancet* 2004;364:613-20.

4 Smoking cessation

Prasima Srivastava, Graeme P Currie, John Britton

Smoking was first introduced into the United Kingdom in the late 16th century. Shortly afterwards, King James I of England implemented the first tax on tobacco use. He also published his famous *A Counterblaste to Tobacco* in 1604, where he reflected on his dislike of the "precious stink" and observed: "Smoking is a custom loathsome to the eye, hateful to the nose, harmful to the brain, dangerous to the lungs, and in the black, stinking fume thereof nearest resembling the horrible Stygian smoke of the pit that is bottomless."

Cigarette smoking delivers nicotine—a powerfully addictive drug—quickly and in high doses directly to the brain. Addiction to nicotine is usually established through experimentation with cigarettes during adolescence and often results in sustained or lifelong smoking. However, nicotine itself does not cause major health problems in most users; it is the accompanying tar that accounts for most of the harm caused by cigarettes.

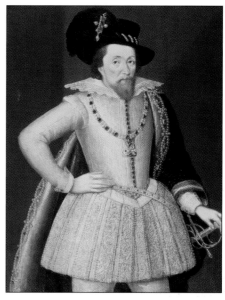

King James I of England, by John de Critz the Elder (c1552-1642). King James I implemented the first tax on tobacco

Effects of cigarette smoking

Apart from being the most common and important cause of chronic obstructive pulmonary disease (COPD), cigarette smoking causes a range of other chronic diseases and cancers affecting almost every bodily system. Cigarette smoking results in more than 100 000 deaths each year in the United Kingdom. Some diseases—including sarcoidosis, extrinsic allergic alveolitis, Parkinson's disease, and ulcerative colitis—are less common in smokers.

Primary prevention of COPD

As long as cigarette smoking remains a normal and acceptable behaviour in adults, preventing children and adolescents from experimenting is difficult. However, measures to reduce children's access to cigarettes will probably help prevent smoking. The most effective approach to primary prevention is the application of general population measures that reduce incentives to smoke in both adults and young people. Examples include

- Comprehensive bans on advertising and promotion
- Sustained increases in real price
- Policing of illegal sources of less expensive cigarettes
- Comprehensive smoke-free policies at work and public places
- Health warnings on cigarette packs
- Sustained health promotion campaigns.

By preventing smoking, all of these measures will reduce the incidence of COPD.

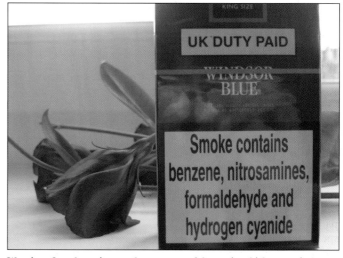

Warnings found on cigarette boxes are useful ways in which to remind individuals of the dangers of smoking

Secondary prevention of COPD

Smoking cessation is the most effective means of secondary prevention for COPD. At any age it reduces disease progression and reduces the rate of decline in lung function in those with established COPD to that of a non-smoker. Individuals with COPD who quit smoking experience a substantial improvement in overall health, functional status, and survival, as well as a reduced incidence of many forms of cancer and cardiovascular diseases. Thus, it is important to emphasise to all patients with COPD that it is never too late to stop smoking.

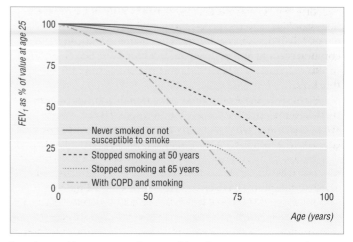

Stopping smoking at any age has beneficial effects on the lung function of patients with COPD

Successful and cost effective smoking cessation interventions have been available for many years. These include generic population measures to encourage smoking cessation (and to discourage uptake of smoking) as mentioned above, plus individual interventions involving behavioural support and pharmacotherapy.

Helping patients stop smoking

Behavioural support

All health professionals should encourage all smokers to quit at every available opportunity. Always offer advice in an encouraging, non-judgmental, and empathetic manner. Explain to patients with COPD who still smoke that stopping is not easy and that several attempts may be required to achieve long term success. Find out if they are motivated to stop and, if so, support a quit attempt as soon as possible.

If they are not motivated, explore their reasons for not quitting and encourage them to consider doing so in the future. Introduce the idea that a cigarette is a killer and should not be regarded as a "comforting friend" in times of anxiety and stress. Explain that cigarette smoking is pleasurable or relaxing primarily because it relieves withdrawal symptoms—remind patients of their first experience of smoking and ask if it was pleasant. List the harmful chemicals and carcinogens that are found in cigarettes (such as benzene and arsenic) and all the diseases that smoking causes.

Highlight the importance of behavioural support and pharmacotherapy, and encourage patients to use both. Discuss potential nicotine withdrawal symptoms and explain that these are at their worst in the first few days and most will pass within about a month. Weight gain is often a concern, so emphasise the need to eat healthily, drink water before meals, and exercise. Formal dietary advice may be necessary for some individuals. Encourage patients to create goals and rewards for themselves, and highlight the financial benefits of stopping smoking. Devise coping mechanisms to use during periods of craving. Give written information to support your advice so that the risks of smoking and the benefits of quitting can be reinforced at home by family members.

Deliver behavioural advice yourself or ask a smoking cessation specialist to do it for you. Arrange to review all patients, either personally or through a smoking cessation specialist, soon after their quit attempt. Use this review to monitor progress, use alternative strategies if necessary, and provide support and encouragement.

Nicotine replacement therapy

Nicotine replacement is the most common drug treatment to help smoking cessation and increases the chances of quitting by about 1.7-fold. It works by supplying nicotine without the toxic components of cigarette smoke. Many smokers believe that nicotine is toxic, so emphasise that nicotine is safe; it is the tar that kills.

Nicotine replacement therapy is available in many different formulations. Although some forms (gum, inhalator, nasal spray, and lozenges) deliver nicotine more quickly than others (transdermal patches), all deliver a lower total dose and deliver it to the brain more slowly than does a cigarette. Since there is no clear evidence that any formulation is more effective than another, the best approach is to follow individual patients' preference over choice of product. For heavy smokers, there is theoretical support for using a combination of a sustained release product (to provide continuous background nicotine) plus a more rapidly acting product in anticipation of, or at times of, craving.

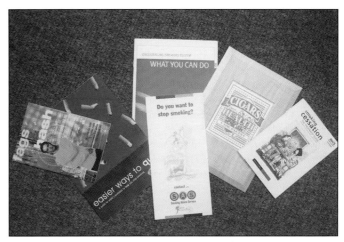

Verbal and written smoking cessation advice should be given to all current smokers at all available opportunities

---

Brief advice on smoking cessation

- Brief advice from health professionals should be given to all smokers. Doing so causes 2-3% of smokers to become long term abstainers and is probably the most cost effective clinical intervention
- "The best thing you can do for your health is to stop smoking, and I advise you to stop as soon as possible. The sooner you stop the better."
- "How do you feel about your smoking?"
- "How do you feel about tackling your smoking now?"

Behavioural strategies for smoking cessation

- Set a quit date and tell friends and colleagues that you are quitting
- Prepare by avoiding smoking in places where you spend a lot of time
- Get rid of all cigarettes
- Don't "cut down" or "have the odd one"—aim for total abstinence
- Review past attempts; look at what has helped and what hasn't
- Anticipate challenges and think of ways of dealing with them
- Encourage partners to quit at the same time and offer them support
- Use nicotine replacement therapy or bupropion
- Make use of follow-up support

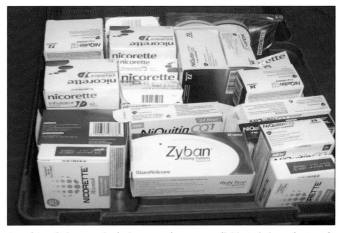

A variety of pharmacological preparations are available to help patients quit smoking

In some smokers with relative contraindications to treatment (such as acute cardiovascular disease or pregnancy) it may be prudent to use low doses of relatively short acting preparations, though in practice nicotine replacement rarely causes problems. Light smokers (< 10 cigarettes a day) and those who wait longer than an hour before their first cigarette of the day may also be best advised to choose a short acting product and to use it in advance of their regular cigarettes or at times of craving.

Nicotine replacement therapy is recommended for up to three months, followed by a gradual withdrawal. The products are generally well tolerated.

Bupropion

Bupropion is of similar efficacy as nicotine replacement in improving quit rates. It is an antidepressant, but its effect on smoking cessation seems to be independent of this property. Like nicotine replacement therapy, bupropion also helps to prevent weight gain. Its main adverse effect is its association with convulsions, and it is therefore contraindicated in patients with a history of epilepsy or seizures. Bupropion should not generally be prescribed for people with other risk factors for seizures, and some drugs—such as antidepressants, antimalarials, antipsychotics, quinolones, and theophylline—can lower the seizure threshold.

Unlike nicotine replacement therapy, which is usually started at the time of quitting smoking, bupropion should be started one or two weeks before the quit date. The initial dose should be 150 mg daily for six days, increasing thereafter to 150 mg twice daily. Stop treatment if the patient has not quit smoking within eight weeks. There is no clear evidence that combining bupropion with nicotine replacement further improves quit rates, and it can lead to hypertension and insomnia.

Other drug treatments

The antidepressant nortriptyline seems to be as effective as nicotine replacement and bupropion as a smoking cessation therapy. Other new treatments are in an advanced stage of clinical trials and may become available in the near future, one of which, varenicline, is a nicotine receptor blocker and partial agonist. There is no evidence that complementary therapies such as hypnosis or acupuncture are effective.

Implementing smoking cessation in routine care

One of the major barriers to smoking cessation practice is that many health professionals do not have the skills and knowledge to intervene, or fail to intervene routinely in clinical practice. It is essential that ascertaining smoking status, delivering brief advice, and offering further help to smokers interested in quitting becomes routine practice throughout all medical disciplines, and especially with patients with COPD.

Stopping smoking is the only effective long term intervention in the management of COPD, but too many patients are still not offered the treatments that could help them quit. All smokers should receive smoking cessation intervention, however brief, at all contacts with their doctor and other health professionals. It is also important to advise patients unable to completely quit, that a reduction in the number of cigarettes smoked may still produce some benefit.

Prescribing points with nicotine replacement therapy

Adverse effects	Cautions
● Nausea	● Hyperthyroidism
● Headache	● Diabetes
● Unpleasant taste	● Renal and hepatic impairment
● Hiccoughs and indigestion	● Gastritis and peptic ulcer disease
● Sore throat	● Peripheral vascular disease
● Nose bleeds	● Skin disorders (patches)
● Palpitations	● Avoid nasal spray when driving or operating machinery (sneezing, watering eyes)
● Dizziness	● Severe cardiovascular disease (arrhythmias, after myocardial infarction)
● Insomnia	● Recent stroke
● Nasal irritation (with spray)	● Pregnancy
	● Breast feeding

Note that, even with many of the cautions above, nicotine replacement therapy is still preferable to continued smoking

---

Contraindications to prescribing bupropion

- History of seizures
- Use of drugs that lower the seizure threshold
- Symptoms of alcohol or benzodiazepine withdrawal
- Eating disorders
- Bipolar illness
- Central nervous system tumours
- Pregnancy
- Breast feeding
- Severe hepatic cirrhosis

The five A's of smoking cessation

These should form a routine component of all health service delivery
- *Ask* about tobacco use
- *Advise* quitting smoking
- *Assess* willingness to make an attempt
- *Assist* in quit attempt
- *Arrange* follow up

Further reading

- Silagy C, Lancaster T, Stead L, Mant D, Fowler G. Nicotine replacement therapy for smoking cessation. *Cochrane Database Syst Rev* 2004;(3):CD000146
- Hughes JR, Stead LF, Lancaster T. Antidepressants for smoking cessation. *Cochrane Database Syst Rev* 2004;(4):CD000031
- Roddy E. Bupropion and other non-nicotine pharmacotherapies. *BMJ* 2004;328:509-11
- Jamrozik K. Population strategies to prevent smoking. *BMJ* 2004; 328:759-62
- Molyneux A. Nicotine replacement therapy. *BMJ* 2004;328:454-6
- West R, McNeill A, Raw M. Smoking cessation guidelines for health professionals: an update. Health Education Authority. *Thorax* 2000; 55:987-99

Competing interests: GPC has received funding for attending international conferences and honoraria for giving talks from pharmaceutical companies GlaxoSmithKline, Pfizer, and AstraZeneca. JB has received an honorarium and travel expenses for speaking at a conference from a manufacturer of nicotine replacement products, has been involved in clinical trials of such products, and has been a paid consultant for companies developing such products.

The portrait of King James I is reproduced with permission of Roy Miles Fine Paintings/BAL. The graph showing the effect of stopping smoking on lung function is adapted from Hogg JC. *Lancet* 2004;364:709-21.

5 Non-pharmacological management

Graeme P Currie, J Graham Douglas

Chronic obstructive pulmonary disease (COPD) is a progressive and largely irreversible disorder. Unsurprisingly, drugs alone cannot ensure optimum short and long term outcomes. As a consequence, there is increasing interest in the role of non-drug strategies and multi-disciplinary team input in the overall management of COPD.

Pulmonary rehabilitation

Depending on local availability, consider referring all COPD patients—irrespective of age, functional limitation, and smoking status—for pulmonary rehabilitation. This is defined as "a multidisciplinary programme of care for patients with chronic respiratory impairment that is individually tailored and designed to optimise physical and social performance and autonomy." A suitable programme is important in breaking the vicious cycle of worsening breathlessness, reduced physical activity, and deconditioning that many patients experience, and pulmonary rehabilitation plays a major role in restoring patients to an optimally functioning state. For example, early intervention after an acute exacerbation of COPD can produce clinically significant improvements in exercise capacity and health. The ideal programme should consist of several components, including exercise training, education, and nutritional support.

Exercise training—Outpatient pulmonary rehabilitation programmes typically run for two months, with two or three sessions of supervised exercise each week. Patients are encouraged to exercise at home and record their achievements, so that progress can be monitored. Studies have shown that physiological changes provided by endurance training take place at the level of skeletal muscle, even during sub-maximal exercise. Exercise training can improve exercise tolerance, symptoms, quality of life, peak oxygen uptake, endurance time during sub-maximal exercise, functional walking distance, and peripheral and respiratory muscle strength.

Education—This generally comprises various forms of goal directed and systematically applied communication aimed at improving understanding and motivation. The programme should be structured, and potential topics include breathing control, relaxation, benefits of exercise, and value of smoking cessation. Although education individualised to the patient is often helpful, group based education may be more effective. Participants are encouraged to take responsibility for their own health, and follow-up sessions may be necessary at home.

Nutritional advice—The term COPD encompasses patients previously labelled as being overweight "blue bloaters" and underweight "pink puffers." Despite the marked differences in body habitus and nutritional status, the pathophysiological hallmark in both phenotypes is relatively fixed airflow obstruction. Many COPD patients are underweight because of the heightened energy output associated with the increased work of breathing and reduced nutritional intake due to limitations posed by severe breathlessness. However, patients can become overweight because of reduced activity and overeating. The reasons for these phenotypic differences are far from clear, but raised concentrations of cytokines such as tumour necrosis factor α and leptin have been implicated in weight loss.

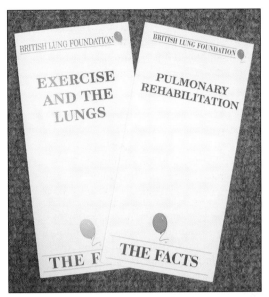

Pulmonary rehabilitation should be offered to most patients with COPD

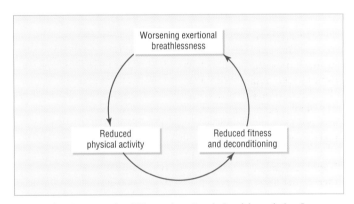

A determined attempt should be made to break the vicious circle of worsening breathlessness, reduced physical activity and deconditioning

---

Nutritional advice for COPD patients

- Calculate the body mass index (weight (kg)/(height (m)^2)) of all patients
- Arrange dietary advice for those who are underweight (index < 18.5) or obese (index > 30), and those whose weight is changing over time

Although these recommendations are not supported by a Cochrane review of the effects of nutritional supplementation in COPD (which failed to show any significant impact on lung function or exercise capacity), the number of double blind studies and participants included in the review were small, and it seems logical to ensure adequate nutritional intake in all patients with chronic disease, including COPD

Long term outcomes of pulmonary rehabilitation
Improved exercise performance and reduced breathlessness associated with exercise can be maintained for up to 12 months. Pulmonary rehabilitation can also improve quality of life, but this benefit tends to decline over time. Moreover, there is no influence on disease progression (as judged by decline in forced expiratory volume in 1 second (FEV_1)), and there is little evidence of improvement in long term survival. Data about use of healthcare resources are conflicting, with no consistent reduction in hospital admission rates or length of hospital stay.

Immunisation

Many exacerbations of COPD are caused by viral and bacterial infection, suggesting that vaccination could reduce the number of exacerbations. Unless they are contraindicated, arrange pneumococcal and influenza immunisation in all patients with COPD.

Pneumococcal vaccination–Current pneumococcal vaccines contain 25 ng of purified capsular polysaccharide from each of 23 subtypes of *Streptococcus pneumoniae*. A single dose of 0.5 ml is given intramuscularly, and mild soreness and induration at the site of injection is common. Re-immunisation is not advised and is contraindicated within three years. The severe reactions to re-immunisations that occur are probably due to high levels of circulating antibodies. Although evidence suggests that the current 23 valent vaccine is effective in preventing the bacteraemia associated with pneumococcal pneumonia, there is no convincing evidence of benefit to patients with COPD.

Influenza vaccination–Influenza vaccine is prepared each year with viruses (usually two type A and one type B) similar to those considered most likely to be circulating in the forthcoming winter. The viruses are grown in the allantoic cavity of chick embryos, and the vaccine is therefore contraindicated in people with egg allergy. Patients are often concerned about adverse effects, and doubts may exist about the protective effects of the vaccine. A Cochrane review of 20 cohort studies evaluating the effects of inactivated influenza vaccine in high risk patients (including some with COPD) confirmed that vaccination did confer an overall reduction in exacerbation rates. In another meta-analysis of patients given influenza vaccination, the pooled estimates of efficacy for patients older than 65 years were 56% for preventing respiratory illness, 53% for preventing pneumonia, 50% for preventing hospital admission, and 68% for preventing death.

Mental health status

Many patients with COPD have anxiety and depression, which are likely to further impair quality of life. These conditions are probably multifactorial in origin, with social isolation, persistent symptoms, and inability to participate in many activities of daily living all likely to play a role. Positively search for features suggestive of an anxiety or depressive disorder. Mental health status can be assessed with simple tools such as the hospital anxiety and depression scale. If anxiety or depression is present, treat with conventional drugs, although care should be taken with the use of benzodiazepines and other respiratory depressants. Common sense also suggests that an aggressive attempt to optimise lung function and improve substantial hypoxaemia should be undertaken in these patients.

Surgery

Many COPD patients are unsuitable for surgical intervention because of high operative risk, and careful consideration is

---

Overall aims of treatment of COPD
- Reduce symptoms
- Improve exercise tolerance
- Improve health related quality of life
- Prevent exacerbations
- Provide package of care that meets the patient's needs
- Provide treatment that minimises the risk of adverse effects
- Reduce mortality
- Prevent disease progression

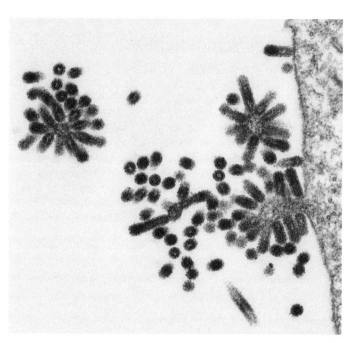

Electron micrograph showing influenza viruses (red) budding from a host cell

---

Hospital anxiety and depression scale

Scoring is based on a 4 point scale (0-3). A score of 0-7 is normal, 8-10 borderline, and 11-21 suggests moderate to severe anxiety or depression

Anxiety
- I feel tense or wound up (Most of the time (3) to Not at all (0))
- I get sort of frightened feelings as if something awful is going to happen (Definitely and badly (3) to Not at all (0))
- Worrying thoughts go through my mind (Definitely (3) to Not at all (0))
- I can sit at ease and feel relaxed (Definitely (0) to Not at all (3))
- I get a sort of frightened feeling like butterflies in the stomach (Not at all (0) to Very often (3))
- I feel restless as if I have to be on the move (Very much (3) to Not at all (0))
- I get sudden feelings of panic (Very often (3) to Not at all (0))

Depression
- I look forward with enjoyment to things (As much as I ever did (0) to Hardly at all (3))
- I have lost interest in my appearance (Definitely (3) to I take as much care as ever (0))
- I still enjoy the things I used to enjoy (Definitely as much (0) to Hardly at all (3))
- I can laugh and see the funny side of things (As much as I always could (0) to Not at all (3))
- I feel cheerful (Not at all (3) to Most of the time (0))
- I feel as if I am slowed down (Nearly all the time (3) to Not at all (0))
- I can enjoy a good book, the radio, or a TV programme (Often (0) to Seldom (3))

required before contemplating a procedure. The three most common procedures—bullectomy, lung volume reduction surgery, and transplantation—carry substantial short and long term risks of morbidity and mortality. They are therefore generally limited to motivated former smokers who have serious symptoms despite maximal treatment.

Bullectomy—In some patients with COPD, bullae can occupy large volumes of the thoracic cavity, causing compression of surrounding functional lung parenchyma. Bullectomy should be considered in symptomatic patients with a large bulla—especially those with moderate or severe airflow obstruction, a prior pneumothorax, or haemoptysis. Differentiating a pneumothorax from a large lung bulla can be difficult, and computed tomography of the chest may be required. Inadvertent insertion of a chest drain into a bulla can lead to complications such as the development of a bronchopleural fistula.

Lung volume reduction surgery—Lung volume reduction surgery involves removal of segments of inefficient emphysematous lung parenchyma in order to promote better gas exchange in the remaining, less affected part. The procedure can improve quality of life, exercise capacity, and lung function in carefully selected individuals, and, in subgroup analysis in some studies, prolong survival. Moreover, it is a safer procedure than lung transplantation and avoids the problem of lack of donor lungs. Consider surgical referral of patients fulfilling the criteria of predominantly upper lobe disease, markedly impaired exercise capacity despite appropriate treatment, and $FEV_1 > 20\%$ of the predicted value. Recently, interest has been growing in bronchoscopic lung volume reduction in patients with COPD. This involves obstructing emphysematous areas of lung with, for example, an endobronchial valve—therefore avoiding the risks associated with major surgery. The potential role of this procedure in treating COPD requires further evaluation.

Lung transplantation—Some motivated former smokers with COPD should be considered for lung transplantation, although, as in most transplant procedures, this is greatly limited by organ availability. Patients with concomitant medical conditions and advanced age generally have poor survival rates. The upper age limit is generally considered to be 60 years for a bilateral lung transplant, and 65 years for a single lung transplant. Local guidelines should be consulted, but suggested criteria for referral include patients with a combination of advanced airflow obstruction, significant functional impairment, cor pulmonale, and life expectancy of less than two years.

Multidisciplinary care

Members of a multidisciplinary team can greatly assist patients with the physical, domestic, and social limitations imposed by severe breathlessness. Respiratory nurse specialists are likely to have an increasingly important role and can provide a vital interface between primary and secondary care. Areas where they can provide support include helping patients deal with emotional and psychological sequelae, patient education, assessing inhaler technique, nebuliser assessments, nurse prescribing, organisation of assisted discharge schemes, monitoring domiciliary non-invasive ventilation, and end of life palliation and family support.

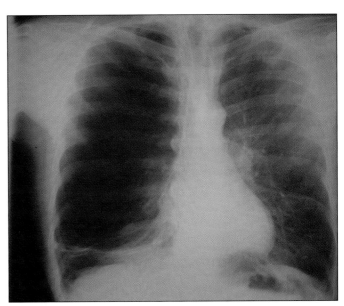

A large right sided lung bulla in a patient with COPD

Multidisciplinary team members often required for optimal care of patients with COPD

- Hospital doctors
- General practitioners
- Respiratory nurse specialists
- Social workers
- Dietians
- Occupational therapists
- Pharmacists
- Mental health care workers
- Physiotherapists

Further reading

- British Thoracic Society guidelines. Pulmonary rehabilitation. *Thorax* 2001;56:827-34
- Man WD, Polkey MI, Donaldson N, Gray BJ, Moxham J. Community pulmonary rehabilitation after hospitalisation for acute exacerbations of chronic obstructive pulmonary disease: randomised controlled study. *BMJ* 2004;329:1209-11
- Gross PA, Hermogenes AW, Sacks HS, Lau J, Levandowski RA. The efficacy of influenza vaccine in elderly persons. A meta-analysis and review of the literature. *Ann Intern Med* 1995;123:518-27
- Poole PJ, Chacko E, Wood-Baker RWB, Cates CJ. Influenza vaccine for patients with chronic obstructive pulmonary disease. *Cochrane Database Syst Rev* 2000;(4):CD002733
- Ferreira IM, Brooks D, Lacasse Y, Goldstein RS. Nutritional support for individuals with COPD: a meta-analysis. *Chest* 2000;117:672-8
- Fishman A, Martinez F, Naunheim K, Piantadosi S, Wise R, Ries A, et al. A randomized trial comparing lung-volume-reduction surgery with medical therapy for severe emphysema. *N Engl J Med* 2003;348:2059-73
- Hopkinson NS, Toma TP, Hansell DM, Goldstraw P, Moxham J, Geddes DM, et al. Effect of bronchoscopic lung volume reduction on dynamic hyperinflation and exercise in emphysema. *Am J Respir Crit Care Med* 2005;171:453-60

Competing interests: GPC has received funding for attending international conferences and honoraria for giving talks from pharmaceutical companies GlaxoSmithKline, Pfizer, and AstraZeneca. JGD has received funding for attending international conferences from GlaxoSmithKline and Novartis; fees for speaking from Boehringer, AstraZeneca, Atlanta, and GlaxoSmithKline; and research funding from Boehringer and GlaxoSmithKline.

The electron micrograph of influenza virus is reproduced with permission of Steve Gschmeissner and Science Photo Library.

6 Pharmacological management—inhaled treatment

Graeme P Currie, Brian J Lipworth

Chronic obstructive airways disease (COPD) is a heterogeneous condition, and all patients should be viewed as individuals—not only in terms of presentation, history, symptoms, and disability, but also in response to treatment. Acceptability to the patient, possible adverse effects, and efficacy of treatment are important factors to consider when prescribing inhaled drugs. The titration of drug treatment in COPD is usually based on the degree of airflow obstruction, severity of symptoms, exercise tolerance, and frequency of exacerbations.

Short acting bronchodilators

For all patients with established COPD, prescribe a short acting inhaled bronchodilator (β_2 agonist or anticholinergic, or both in combination).

Short acting β_2 agonists such as salbutamol reduce breathlessness and improve lung function, and are effective when used "as required." They act directly on bronchial smooth muscle and cause the airways to dilate for up to six hours.

Short acting anticholinergics such as ipratropium reduce breathlessness, improve lung function, improve health related quality of life, and reduce the need for rescue medication. They offset high resting bronchomotor tone and improve airway calibre for up to six hours.

Both drugs in combination (salbutamol plus ipratropium delivered via a metered dose inhaler) have been shown to confer greater improvement in lung function than either drug given alone.

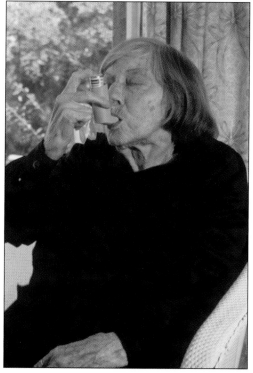

All patients with established COPD should be prescribed a short acting inhaled bronchodilator for use as required

Long acting bronchodilators

For patients with persistent symptoms and exacerbations, prescribe a long acting bronchodilator. Current guidelines recommend monotherapy with a long acting β_2 agonist or anticholinergic for symptomatic patients with mild airflow obstruction (forced expiratory volume in 1 second (FEV_1) 50-80% of predicted value).

Inhaled long acting bronchodilators confer important clinical benefits beyond changes in FEV_1. Therefore, relying on measures of lung function alone to monitor the effects of bronchodilators may miss important physiological and clinical benefits. Air trapping, which is manifest clinically as hyperinflation, often occurs in advanced COPD and places the respiratory muscles at mechanical disadvantage. During exercise, air trapping increases even further, perpetuating the mechanical disadvantage experienced at rest. Long acting bronchodilators often reduce measures of air trapping at rest and on exercise (static and dynamic hyperinflation), and these may well occur without significant changes in FEV_1.

Long acting ß₂ agonists

β_2 agonists act directly on β_2 adrenoceptors, causing smooth muscle to relax and airways to dilate. The two most widely used long acting drugs—formoterol and salmeterol—have a duration of action of at least 12 hours and therefore are indicated for twice daily use. In contrast to the short acting β_2 agonists, these drugs are relatively lipophilic (fat soluble) and have prolonged receptor occupancy. Factors such as these may in part explain

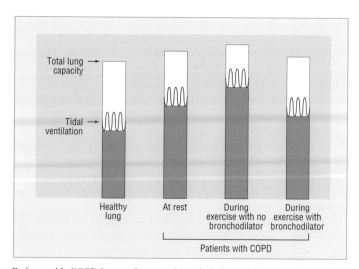

Patients with COPD have pulmonary hyperinflation, with increased functional residual capacity (red) and decreased inspiratory capacity (white). This increases the volume at which tidal breathing (oscillating line) occurs and places the respiratory muscles at mechanical disadvantage. Hyperinflation worsens with exercise and reduces exercise tolerance (dynamic hyperinflation). Inhaled bronchodilators improve dynamic hyperinflation and hyperinflation at rest, reducing the work of breathing and increasing exercise tolerance

their prolonged duration of action. In vitro data have shown that formoterol relaxes smooth muscle more potently than does salmeterol, and it has a much quicker onset of action, similar to that of the short acting β$_2$ agonist salbutamol.

Regular use of a long acting β$_2$ agonist by patients with COPD generally leads to improved lung function, symptoms, and quality of life. A Cochrane systematic review of eight trials evaluating the effects of these drugs on COPD found inconsistent effects on exacerbations.

Long acting anticholinergics
The characteristic airflow obstruction in COPD is multifactorial in origin and is partially due to potentially reversible high cholinergic tone. Furthermore, mechanisms mediated by the vagus nerve are implicated in the enhanced secretion by submucosal glands seen in patients with COPD. This knowledge has led to the development of a long acting anticholinergic taken once daily (tiotropium), which is likely to supersede short acting drugs (ipratropium and oxitropium).

Three main subtypes of muscarinic receptor exist (M$_1$, M$_2$, and M$_3$). Activation of the M$_1$ and M$_3$ receptors results in bronchoconstriction, whereas the M$_2$ receptor is protective against such an effect. In contrast to ipratropium, tiotropium dissociates rapidly from the M$_2$ receptor (therefore minimising the loss of any putative benefit) and dissociates only slowly from the M$_3$ receptor. This prolongs the reduction in resting bronchomotor tone, smooth muscle relaxation, and airway dilation. Tiotropium's onset of peak bronchodilation is between one and three hours. It is the only long acting anticholinergic currently licensed in the United Kingdom and is delivered to the airways via a breath activated, dry powder inhaler at a dose of 18 µg/day. With this device, tiotropium can be successfully deposited in the airways of patients with very low inspiratory flow rates.

Many studies of patients with COPD have shown tiotropium to be more effective than ipratropium (and placebo) in terms of lung function, symptoms, quality of life and exacerbations. Few studies have directly compared tiotropium with long acting β$_2$ agonists, but in one study tiotropium was better than salmeterol at improving lung function. Further investigations are needed to clarify the place of tiotropium in treating patients with COPD of varying severity and how it compares with other inhaled treatments.

Inhaled corticosteroids
Commonly prescribed inhaled corticosteroids include beclometasone dipropionate, budesonide, and fluticasone propionate. Many patients with COPD, even those with minimal symptoms and mild airflow obstruction, have been traditionally treated with inhaled corticosteroids as monotherapy. This is despite corticosteroids' relative ineffectiveness on the neutrophilic inflammation found in COPD and lack of evidence of significant short or long term benefits. Historically, this was due to clinicians incorrectly extending the beneficial role of anti-inflammatory treatment in asthma to COPD, plus a lack of alternative drug treatments.

The exact role of inhaled corticosteroids in the management of COPD is uncertain. It is fairly well established that, as monotherapy, they do not have any appreciable impact on the rate of decline in FEV$_1$ or in improving survival. In one large study (ISOLDE), 1000 µg/day of fluticasone did confer a 25% reduction in exacerbations, with most benefit being observed in patients with mean FEV$_1$ < 50% of predicted. Other studies have shown inconsistent effects on secondary end points, with no or only small improvements in symptoms and quality of life.

Adverse effects of long acting bronchodilators
Although long acting β$_2$ agonists and anticholinergics are generally well tolerated, adverse effects do occur in a minority of patients.

β$_2$ agonists	**Anticholinergics**
● Tachycardia	● Dry mouth
● Fine tremor	● Nausea
● Headache	● Constipation
● Muscle cramps	● Headache
● Prolongation of QT interval	● Tachycardia
● Hypokalaemia	● Acute angle glaucoma
● Feeling of nervousness	● Bladder outflow obstruction

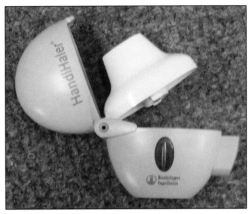

Breath activated inhaler device used to deliver tiotropium to the endobronchial tree

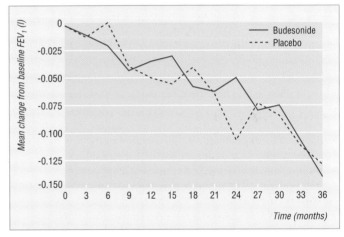

Effect of inhaled corticosteroid (budesonide) on rate of decline in lung function of patients with mild COPD: compared with placebo, corticosteroid made no difference in mean change in baseline FEV$_1$ over 36 months

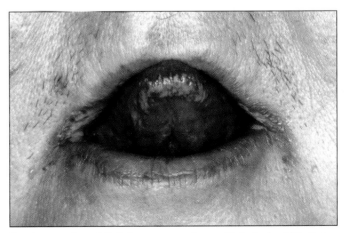

Oropharyngeal candidiasis is a common adverse effect of using high dose inhaled corticosteroids

The dose of inhaled corticosteroid required to achieve maximal beneficial effect with minimal adverse effect (optimum therapeutic ratio) is uncertain, and more data are needed. As a consequence, consider prescribing regular, high dose, inhaled corticosteroids in patients with an FEV_1 <50% of predicted and who experience frequent exacerbations (>2 a year).

Combined corticosteroid plus long acting β₂ agonist inhalers

Using a long acting β₂ agonist combined with a corticosteroid in a single inhaler device—such as Symbicort (budesonide plus formoterol) and Seretide (fluticasone plus salmeterol)—is more convenient than taking the drugs separately. This facilitates compliance by patients with more severe airflow obstruction and frequent exacerbations, who require both drugs. Studies have shown that the combination product is often more effective than the individual component as monotherapy, although in all of these studies the mean FEV_1 was <50% of predicted. Trials of combination inhalers for patients with less severe airflow obstruction are required to establish their role fully. The role of "triple therapy" (corticosteroid and long acting β₂ agonist combination inhaler plus long acting anticholinergic) in more severe disease also needs to be defined.

Summary of inhaled treatment

Since airflow obstruction is the universal feature of clinically significant COPD, bronchodilators play an integral role in all stages of disease. All patients with symptomatic COPD need a short acting inhaled bronchodilator for use "as required," while those with mild airflow obstruction (FEV_1 50-80% of predicted) should regularly use a long acting bronchodilator. In other words, patients with persistent symptoms despite intermittent use of a short acting bronchodilator should use a long acting β₂ agonist twice daily or a long acting anticholinergic once daily as first line treatment. Guidelines do not suggest which class of long acting bronchodilator should be used in the first instance.

If symptoms persist despite use of a long acting bronchodilator, prescribe both classes of long acting bronchodilator concomitantly to maximally dilate the airways. Inhaled corticosteroids play less of a role in COPD management and should be reserved for patients with more advanced airflow obstruction (FEV_1 <50% of predicted) and frequent exacerbations. Consider prescribing "triple therapy" with all three classes of inhaled drug in those with persistent symptoms, exacerbations, and severe airflow obstruction.

Competing interests: GPC has received funding for attending international conferences and honoraria for giving talks from pharmaceutical companies GlaxoSmithKline, Pfizer, and AstraZeneca. BJL has received funding for attending conferences, payment for speaking and consulting activity, and research funding from pharmaceutical companies AstraZeneca, Atlanta, Aerocrine, Sepracor, MSD, Neolab, Cipla, Innovata, UCB-Celltech, and Schering-Plough.

The picture of an elderly patient using an inhaler was supplied by Mark Clarke and Science Photo Library. The diagram of the effects of bronchodilators on hyperinflation was adapted from Sutherland et al. *N Engl J Med* 2004;350:2689-97. The graph of the effect of budesonide on rate of lung function decline was adapted from Vestbo et al. *Lancet* 1999;353:1819-23.

Adverse effects of inhaled corticosteroids

- Inhaled corticosteroids can cause both local and systemic adverse effects
- Common local effects include oropharyngeal candidiasis and dysphonia. Using a spacer device and rinsing the mouth and brushing teeth after using an inhaled corticosteroid can reduce the risk of these problems
- Systemic effects include an increased tendency to skin bruising and, possibly, reduction of bone mineral density and suppression of the hypothalamic-pituitary-adrenal axis

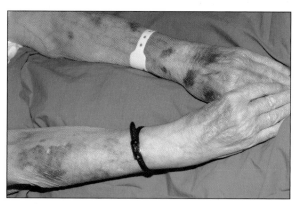

Extensive skin bruising in a patient using high dose inhaled corticosteroids

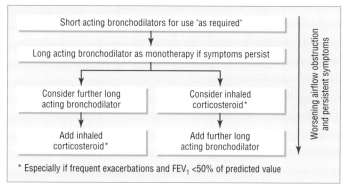

Algorithm for inhaled drug treatment in patients with COPD

Further reading

- National clinical guideline on management of chronic obstructive pulmonary disease in adults in primary and secondary care. *Thorax* 2004;59(suppl 1):1-232
- Pauwels RA, Buist AS, Calverley PM, Jenkins CR, Hurd SS. Global strategy for the diagnosis, management, and prevention of chronic obstructive pulmonary disease. NHLBI/WHO Global Initiative for Chronic Obstructive Lung Disease (GOLD) workshop summary. *Am J Respir Crit Care Med* 2001;163:1256-76
- Celli BR, MacNee W. Standards for the diagnosis and treatment of patients with COPD: a summary of the ATS/ERS position paper. *Eur Respir J* 2004;23:932-46
- Appleton S, Poole P, Smith B, Veale A, Bara A. Long-acting β₂-agonists for chronic obstructive pulmonary disease patients with poorly reversible airflow limitation. *Cochrane Database Syst Rev* 2002;(3):CD001104
- Currie GP, Rossiter C, Miles SA, Lee DKC, Dempsey OJ. Effects of tiotropium and other long acting bronchodilators in chronic obstructive pulmonary disease. *Pulm Pharmacol Ther* 2006;19:112-9
- Burge PS, Calverley PM, Jones PW, Spencer S, Anderson JA, Maslen TK. Randomised, double blind, placebo controlled study of fluticasone propionate in patients with moderate to severe chronic obstructive pulmonary disease: the ISOLDE trial. *BMJ* 2000;320: 1297-303
- Lung Health Study Research Group. Effect of inhaled triamcinolone on the decline in pulmonary function in chronic obstructive pulmonary disease. *N Engl J Med* 2000;343:1902-9

7 Pharmacological management—oral treatment

Graeme P Currie, Daniel K C Lee, Brian J Lipworth

Inhaled treatment forms the cornerstone of drug management of chronic obstructive pulmonary disease (COPD). However, some patients—especially those who are elderly, cognitively impaired, or with upper limb musculoskeletal problems—are unable to use inhaler devices successfully.

Theophylline

Theophylline is one of the oldest oral bronchodilators available for the treatment of COPD. It has a similar chemical structure to caffeine, which is also a bronchodilator in large amounts.

Theophylline is a non-selective phosphodiesterase inhibitor, and it causes an increase in the intracellular concentration of cyclic AMP in various cell types and organs (including the lung). Increased cyclic AMP concentrations are implicated in inhibition of inflammatory and immunomodulatory cells. One result is that phosphodiesterase inhibition causes smooth muscle relaxation and airway dilation.

Other potentially beneficial mechanisms of action of theophylline in COPD have been suggested, including
- Reduction of diaphragmatic muscle fatigue
- Increased mucociliary clearance
- Respiratory centre stimulation
- Inhibition of neutrophilic inflammation
- Suppression of inflammatory genes by activation of histone deacetylases
- Inhibition of cytokines and other inflammatory cell mediators
- Potentiation of anti-inflammatory effects of inhaled corticosteroids
- Potentiation of bronchodilator effects of β_2 agonists.

Clinical use of theophylline

Consider a long acting theophylline preparation in patients with advanced COPD, especially when symptoms persist despite the use of inhaled long acting bronchodilators or in patients unable to use inhaler devices. Studies have shown that theophylline generally confers modest benefits in lung function when combined with different classes of inhaled bronchodilators (anticholinergics and β_2 agonists). In a meta-analysis of 20 randomised controlled trials, theophylline conferred some improvement in lung function and arterial blood gas tensions compared with placebo, although the incidence of nausea was significantly higher with the active drug.

The slow onset of action of theophylline combined with the need to titrate the dose to achieve suitable plasma levels mean that most benefit may not be observed until after several weeks. Clinical efficacy should be assessed according to improvements in a variety of end points, such as lung function, symptoms, exacerbations, exercise capacity, quality of life, and patient tolerability and acceptability. As with most drugs for COPD, clinicians should stop treatment if a therapeutic trial is unsuccessful.

Adverse effects

One of the main limitations preventing more extensive use of theophylline is its tendency to cause adverse effects. In addition, several patient characteristics and commonly prescribed drugs alter its half life in the body. Target levels are 10-20 mg/l

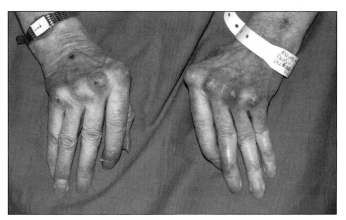

Some patients may not have the manual dexterity required to use hand held inhaler devices. Unfortunately, there are significant unmet needs in terms of effective, long acting, oral bronchodilators for COPD

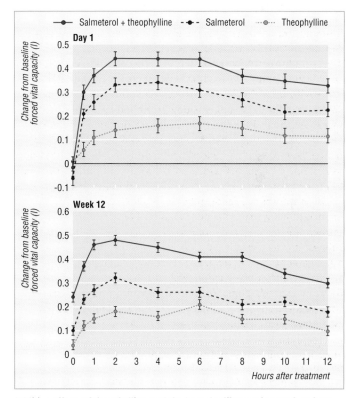

Additive effects of theophylline and the bronchodilator salmeterol on lung function in patients with COPD at day 1 and at 12 weeks after starting treatment

Adverse effects of theophylline

- Tachycardia
- Cardiac arrhythmias
- Nausea and vomiting
- Abdominal pain
- Diarrhoea
- Headache
- Irritability and insomnia
- Seizures
- Hypokalaemia

(55-110 µM), and at higher concentrations the frequency of adverse effects tends to increase to an unacceptable extent.

Explain to patients that it may be necessary to titrate the dose of theophylline slowly upwards until a stable therapeutic level is achieved. During an exacerbation of COPD, reduce the theophylline dose by 50% if a macrolide (such as erythromycin) or fluoroquinolone (such as ciprofloxacin) is prescribed. Selective phosphodiesterase 4 inhibitors have recently been developed with the aim of retaining the beneficial properties of theophylline but avoiding its unwanted effects. The most clinically advanced of these inhibitors are roflumilast and cilomilast, and they show a superior adverse effect and pharmacokinetic profile compared with theophylline.

Oral corticosteroids

Oral corticosteroids have only a limited role in the management of stable COPD, and few data suggest which patients (if any) derive benefit from long term use. Indeed, they have been shown to increase mortality in patients with advanced disease in a dose dependant manner. Prolonged treatment with prednisolone should generally be avoided, although guidelines acknowledge that for some severely affected patients with advanced airflow obstruction it is difficult to stop corticosteroids after an exacerbation. However, this difficulty may in part be due to their mood enhancing effects. When complete withdrawal is impossible, long term use should be limited to the lowest possible dose (such as 5 mg/day of prednisolone).

Managing corticosteroids' adverse effects

Before starting treatment with oral corticosteroids, ensure that patients are aware of the dose to be taken, the anticipated duration, and potential adverse effects. Explain to patients receiving long term oral corticosteroids that treatment should not be stopped suddenly and that the dose must be reduced slowly. Immediate withdrawal after prolonged administration may lead to acute adrenal insufficiency and even death. Issue all patients receiving oral corticosteroids with a treatment card alerting others to the problems associated with abrupt discontinuation. Courses of oral corticosteroids that last less than three weeks (such as for an exacerbation of COPD) do not generally need to be tapered before stopping.

The risk of corticosteroid induced osteoporosis is related to cumulative dose. This means that patients who frequently require short courses of corticosteroid, as well as those taking long term maintenance treatment, may experience this complication. Patients taking ≥ 7.5 mg/day of prednisolone (or equivalent) for three months are at heightened risk of adverse effects, as are those older than 65 years.

Bisphosphonates reduce the rate of bone turnover and are therefore useful in limiting corticosteroid related osteoporosis. Dual emission x ray absorptiometry (DEXA) can facilitate early identification of patients at risk of osteoporosis and are often requested for patients attending specialist clinics. DEXA scans also highlight which patients should ensure adequate dietary intake of calcium and vitamin D3 and, where necessary, start taking weekly bisphosphonate (such as risedronate or alendronate). Patients aged more than 65 years and those who have previously sustained a low velocity fracture should receive bisphosphonate treatment, irrespective of bone density, if they are to use oral corticosteroids on a long term basis.

Mucolytics

Sputum overproduction is common in patients with COPD. Oral mucolytics are thought to reduce the viscosity of sputum

---

Drugs and patient characteristics that affect plasma theophylline concentrations

Increased concentrations (reduced plasma clearance)	Reduced concentrations (increased plasma clearance)
● Heart failure	● Cigarette smoking
● Liver cirrhosis	● Chronic alcoholism
● Advanced age	● Rifampicin
● Ciprofloxacin	● Phenytoin
● Erythromycin	● Carbamazepine
● Clarithromycin	● Lithium
● Verapamil	

Adverse effects of oral corticosteroids

Neuropsychological
- Depression
- Euphoria
- Paranoia
- Insomnia
- Psychological dependence

Musculoskeletal
- Osteoporosis
- Proximal myopathy
- Tendon rupture

Endocrine and metabolic
- Hyperglycaemia
- Hypokalaemia
- Salt and water retention
- Adrenal suppression
- Weight gain
- Menstrual disturbance
- Increased appetite

Skin
- Purple striae
- Moon face
- Acne
- Hirsuitism
- Thin skin and easy bruising

Gastrointestinal
- Peptic ulceration
- Dyspepsia
- Pancreatitis

Ophthalmic
- Cataracts
- Glaucoma
- Papilloedema

Other
- Immunosuppression
- Hypertension
- Neutrophilia

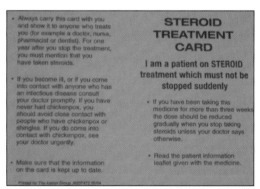

All patients receiving oral corticosteroids should carry a treatment card at all times

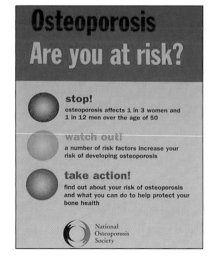

Patients taking frequent courses of oral corticosteroids, or long term maintenance treatment, should be aware of the risks of osteoporosis. They should ensure an adequate intake of dietary calcium and take regular exercise. Postmenopausal women should consider using hormone replacement therapy

in the airways and help patients expectorate. Despite these drugs having no effect on lung function, some studies have found that their regular use reduces the frequency of exacerbations of COPD and is associated with fewer days of ill health.

Two mucolytic agents are currently licensed for use in the United Kingdom (carbocisteine and mecysteine hydrochloride) and are generally well tolerated. They may be tried in patients with productive cough who are troubled by frequent exacerbations, although further data are required to clarify their place in COPD management. Increased oxidative stress has been implicated in the inflammatory response in COPD, and N-acetyl cysteine, another mucolytic, may confer some benefit in terms of its antioxidant properties.

Other drugs

There are no convincing data that prophylactic antibiotics are of use in stable COPD. Indeed, such treatment may only encourage the emergence of strains of bacteria resistant to conventional antibiotics. Cough is a troublesome symptom in many patients, but it may be advantageous, especially in individuals who produce copious amounts of sputum. Cough suppressants are not known to provide any benefit other than perhaps short term symptomatic control of cough, and their regular use is not indicted.

In patients with cor pulmonale there is little evidence that drugs such as angiotensin converting enzyme inhibitors, digoxin, or calcium channel blockers are of any benefit. However, if measures such as leg elevation and, where appropriate, long term oxygen therapy fail to control symptomatic peripheral oedema, low dose diuretics can be tried.

Further reading

- Rennard SI. Treatment of stable chronic obstructive pulmonary disease. *Lancet* 2004;364:791-802
- Ram FSF, Jones PW, Castro AA, de Brito Jardim JR, Atallah AN, Lacasse Y, et al. Oral theophylline for chronic obstructive pulmonary disease. *Cochrane Database Syst Rev* 2002;(4):CD003902
- Barnes PJ. Theophylline: new perspectives on an old drug. *Am J Respir Crit Care Med* 2003;167:813–8
- Lipworth BJ. Phosphodiesterase-4 inhibitors for asthma and chronic obstructive pulmonary disease. *Lancet* 2005;365:167-75
- Poole PJ, Black PN. Oral mucolytic drugs for exacerbations of chronic obstructive pulmonary disease: systematic review. *BMJ* 2001;322: 1271-4

Competing interests: GPC has received funding for attending international conferences and honoraria for giving talks from pharmaceutical companies GlaxoSmithKline, Pfizer, and AstraZeneca. BJL has received funding for attending conferences, payment for speaking and consulting activity, and research funding from pharmaceutical companies AstraZeneca, Atlanta, Aerocrine, Sepracor, MSD, Neolab, Cipla, Innovata, UCB-Celltech, and Schering-Plough.

The figure of the additive effects of theophylline and salmeterol was reproduced with permission from Zu Wallack et al. *Chest* 2001;119: 1661-70.

8 Oxygen and inhalers

Graeme P Currie, J Graham Douglas

Oxygen

Administering oxygen for chronic obstructive pulmonary disease (COPD) is not without risk and it should be properly prescribed—in terms of flow rate and mode of delivery—like any other drug. Giving high concentrations of oxygen to hypoxaemic patients with hypercapnia can result in individuals losing their hypoxic drive to breathe, with development of CO_2 retention, respiratory acidosis, and even death.

However, in acute and chronic ventilatory failure, oxygen supplementation is essential to maintain adequate delivery of oxyhaemoglobin to organs such as the heart, kidneys, and brain. Many patients who are chronically hypoxic are able to cope satisfactorily with an oxygen saturation of arterial blood of around 90%. However, at saturations below this, the oxygen dissociation curve rapidly steepens, and a sharp fall in oxygenated haemoglobin occurs with reduction in oxygen supply to vital organs.

Oxygen during an exacerbation of COPD

During an exacerbation of COPD, give 24% or 28% oxygen via a Venturi facemask to patients with hypercapnia in order to maintain an oxygen saturation >90%. In patients without hypercapnia, titrate the oxygen concentration upwards to keep the saturation >90%. Check arterial blood gases at 30-60 minutes later to check for any rise in CO_2. Nasal cannulas deliver less reliable fractions of inspired oxygen than a facemask but allow patients to communicate, eat, and drink more easily.

Long term oxygen therapy

Two large trials have shown that using oxygen for at least 15 hours a day improves survival of hypoxaemic patients with COPD. Consider long term oxygen therapy in non-smoking patients with COPD if
● Arterial oxygen partial pressure (PaO_2) is <7.3 kPa on two separate occasions at least three weeks apart during a period of clinical stability *or*
● PaO_2 is 7.3-8.0 kPa and there is evidence of secondary polycythaemia, pulmonary hypertension, peripheral oedema, or nocturnal hypoxaemia.

Survival benefits have not been observed in patients who are not sufficiently hypoxaemic or who do not use oxygen for the required length of time each day (≥ 15 hours). Before arranging long term oxygen therapy, ensure that patients have stopped smoking and are aware of the dangers of naked flames near oxygen supplies. Oxygen is most conveniently and economically supplied by a concentrator, which removes nitrogen and therefore produces oxygen-enriched air. Nasal cannulas are the most practical means of delivering oxygen, although some patients—especially those with troublesome drying of the nasal mucosa—may prefer a Venturi facemask.

Short burst oxygen

Despite maximal inhaled and oral drug treatment, many patients with advanced COPD remain breathless on exertion. Such patients are frequently prescribed oxygen cylinders for use "as required." However, studies of oxygen therapy after exercise have failed to show any consistent effect on

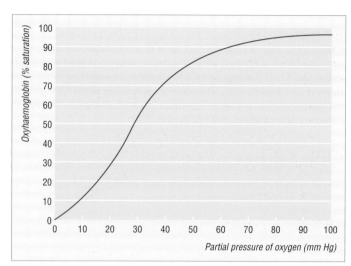

The oxyhaemoglobin dissociation curve showing the relation between partial pressure of oxygen and haemoglobin saturation

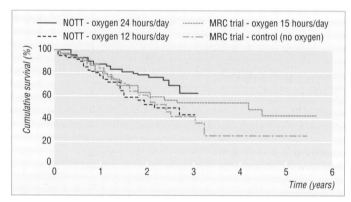

Long term oxygen therapy prolongs survival in hypoxaemic patients with COPD when used for ≥15 hours/day. (Results from the nocturnal oxygen therapy trial (NOTT) and the MRC trial)

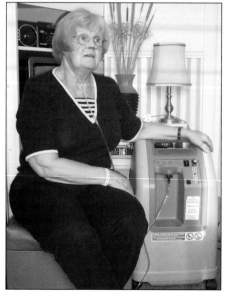

A concentrator supplies oxygen to patients without the need for gas cylinders

breathlessness scores or rate of symptomatic recovery, but it has been shown to reduce the degree of dynamic hyperinflation during recovery from exercise. The potential role of "short burst" oxygen therapy in COPD thus remains controversial, but it should be considered in patients with episodes of severe breathlessness not relieved by other treatments.

Ambulatory oxygen

Patients already receiving long term oxygen therapy can be provided with portable oxygen for use during exercise and activities of daily living outside the home. Its usefulness is limited by the duration of oxygen supply from portable pulse-dose cylinders. In the future, small lightweight cylinders, oxygen conserving devices, and portable liquid oxygen systems may become available. Further studies are needed to establish whether patients who do not fulfil the criteria for provision of long term oxygen therapy but who show significant oxygen desaturation during exercise would also benefit from ambulatory oxygen.

Air travel and oxygen

The partial pressure of oxygen (PO_2) in the air falls with increasing altitude, which can compound any respiratory difficulties faced by a hypoxaemic patient with COPD. Commercial aircraft are pressurised to a cabin pressure of 8000 feet (2438 metres), at which the PO_2 is roughly equivalent to that of 15% oxygen at sea level. Thus, patients with COPD with adequate oxygen saturation at sea level may find oxygenation falls below desirable levels under aircraft cabin pressure. This desaturation is exacerbated by minimal exercise.

Patients with COPD who are planning to travel by air should have their oxygen saturation measured with a pulse oximeter before flights are booked. This helps determine whether in-flight oxygen will be required. All patients who require in-flight oxygen should inform the relevant airline when booking and should be aware that some airlines charge for this service. The need for oxygen on the ground and while changing flights must also be considered, and many airports can provide wheelchairs for transport to and from aircraft. Advise patients to carry both preventive and reliever inhalers in their hand luggage and that nebulisers may be used on aircraft at the discretion of the cabin crew.

Inhalers

Hand held inhalers are used by most patients to facilitate delivery of drugs to the endobronchial tree. Unfortunately, with all inhalers, a substantial proportion of the drug is deposited in the oropharynx. Some patients—such as those who are elderly, cognitively impaired, or with reduced manual dexterity—have difficulty in using inhaler devices.

Before starting inhaled therapy for COPD patients, instruct them on how to use the inhaler device correctly and, if necessary, switch them to an alternative, more suitable device. Moreover, assessment of inhaler technique should be carried out at every available opportunity, as many patients become less proficient over time. The over-riding factors that determine which type of inhaler should be used include patient preference, ease of use, effectiveness of drug delivery, and cost.

Metered dose inhalers

One of the most common inhaler devices is a pressurised metered dose inhaler. Patients notoriously have difficulty in using such inhalers correctly, which has led to the introduction of a variety of other types of inhaler. Correct use of a metered dose inhaler requires strict adherence to the instructions for use.

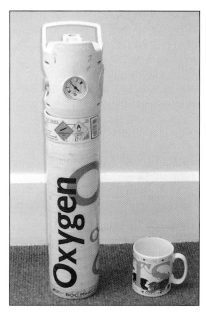

A modern portable cylinder without an oxygen conserving device will last for up to four hours with a flow rate of 2 l/min and up to two hours with a flow rate of 4 l/min

Calculating COPD patients' need for in-flight oxygen in commercial aircraft

Oxygen saturation on air	Recommendation
>95%	Oxygen not required
92-95% (without risk factor*)	Oxygen not required
92-95% (with risk factor*)	Hypoxic challenge test†
<92%	In-flight oxygen required (2 or 4 l/min)
Already using long term oxygen therapy	Increase flow rate

*Risk factors: FEV_1 <50% of predicted, lung cancer, respiratory muscle weakness and other restrictive ventilatory disorders, within 6 weeks of hospital discharge.
†Breathing 15% oxygen at sea level to mimic the reduced PO_2 experienced during a commercial flight. Patients with PaO_2 >7.4 kPa after the challenge do not require in-flight oxygen, those with PaO_2 <6.6 kPa do require oxygen, and those with PaO_2 6.6-7.4 kPa are considered borderline.

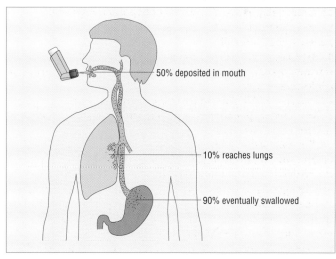

Only a small fraction of drug from a metered dose inhaler reaches the lungs

Correct use of a metered dose inhaler

- Shake the canister
- Take a full breath out (that is, exhale to residual volume)
- Put your lips around the mouthpiece
- Press only once with the inhaler in the mouth and at the same time suck inwards quickly
- Hold your breath for up to 10 seconds
- Breathe out normally

ABC of chronic obstructive pulmonary disease

Metered dose inhaler plus spacer

A spacer device attached to a metered dose inhaler serves two main functions. Firstly, this avoids problems in coordinating the timing of inhaler actuation and inhalation. Secondly, the speed of delivery of the aerosol into the mouth is slowed, which minimises the "cold freon" effect and in turn results in less drug being deposited in the oropharynx and more in the endobronchial tree. If used correctly, a metered dose inhaler with spacer is at least as effective as any other device for delivering inhaled drugs.

Different manufacturers make different sizes of spacers and inhalers, but the following principles of use can applied to most types:
- Shake the inhaler and ensure that it fits snugly into the end of the spacer device
- Place the spacer mouthpiece in the mouth
- Start breathing in and out slowly and gently
- Press the inhaler and continue to breath in and out several more times
- Wait about 30 seconds before repeating the first four steps
- Wipe clean the mouthpiece after use
- Clean the spacer at least once a month with soapy water and leave to air dry
- Replace the spacer every 12 months or according to the manufacturer's recommendations.

Dry powder inhalers

Dry powder inhalers—such as Accuhalers, Turbohalers, Clickhalers, and Twisthalers—are breath activated. They therefore avoid the problem with metered dose inhalers of coordinating inhaler actuation and inhalation. They are also less bulky and more portable. Many patients prefer them to other types of inhaler, but they tend to be more expensive.

Nebulisers

Nebulisers can be driven by oxygen or, for patients with hypercapnic respiratory failure, compressed air. They create a mist of drug particles that are inhaled via a facemask or mouthpiece.

Determining which COPD patients should be prescribed a nebuliser to deliver short acting β_2 agonists and other drugs is controversial. With the introduction of dry powder inhalers, many more patients are now able to use hand held devices correctly, which means that fewer patients need be considered for domiciliary nebulisers. However, it is reasonable to prescribe a nebuliser for patients who remain symptomatic despite maximal treatment with hand held inhalers, although objective evidence of benefit should generally be demonstrated. Patients using a nebuliser should receive adequate training, and be provided with appropriate servicing and support for their equipment from a designated individual.

Competing interests: GPC has received funding for attending international conferences and honorariums for giving talks from pharmaceutical companies GlaxoSmithKline, Pfizer, and AstraZeneca. JGD has received funding for attending international conferences from GlaxoSmithKline and Novartis; fees for speaking from Boehringer, AstraZeneca, Atlanta, and GlaxoSmithKline; and research funding from Boehringer and GlaxoSmithKline.

The graph of the effects of long term oxygen therapy on survival of hypoxaemic patients was adapted from Gorecka et al. *Thorax* 1997;52:674-9

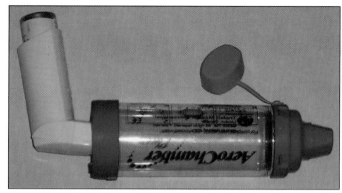

A metered dose inhaler with spacer attached

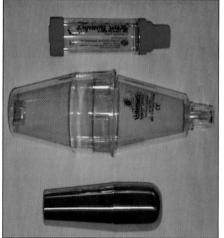

Examples of the various spacer devices produced by different manufacturers

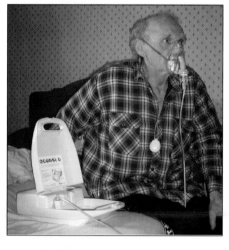

Using a nebuliser is as effective as a metered dose inhaler plus spacer used correctly, and it requires less effort

Further reading

- Bateman NT, Leach RM. ABC of oxygen: Acute oxygen therapy. *BMJ* 1998;317:798-801
- Stevenson NS, Calverley PMA. Effect of oxygen on recovery from maximal exercise in patients with chronic obstructive pulmonary disease. *Thorax* 2004;59:668-72
- Lacasse Y, Laforge J, Maltais F. Got a match? Home oxygen therapy in current smokers. *Thorax* 2006;61:374-5
- Seccombe LM, Kelly PT, Wong CK, Rogers PG, Lim S, Peters MJ. Effect of simulated commercial flight on oxygenation in patients with interstitial lung disease and chronic obstructive pulmonary disease. *Thorax* 2004;59:966-70
- Managing passengers with respiratory disease planning air travel: British Thoracic Society recommendations. *Thorax* 2002;57: 289-304
- BTS guidelines on current best practice for nebuliser treatment. *Thorax* 1997;52(suppl 2):S1-106

9 Acute exacerbations

Graeme P Currie, Jadwiga A Wedzicha

An exacerbation of chronic obstructive pulmonary disease (COPD) is a sustained worsening of respiratory symptoms that is acute in onset and usually requires a patient to seek medical help or alter treatment. The deterioration must be more severe than the usual daily variation experienced. Exacerbations are characterised by increased breathlessness, cough, sputum volume or purulence, wheeze, and chest tightness. Other common features are malaise, reduced exercise tolerance, peripheral oedema, accessory muscle use, confusion, and cyanosis. Other (often coexisting) cardiorespiratory disorders can also cause these symptoms, which may lead to diagnostic uncertainty.

Exacerbations of COPD account for up to 10% of all medical admissions to UK hospitals, equating to more than 100 000 admissions a year, with a mean length of stay of over a week. Exacerbations therefore have considerable costs for secondary care and are partly responsible for high occupancy rates of hospital beds. Patients with frequent exacerbations have an accelerated decline in lung function, impaired quality of life, and restricted daily living activities, and, as a consequence, are likely to become housebound. As the disease becomes more severe, the frequency of exacerbations also increases.

Causes

Exacerbations of COPD are mainly caused by viruses, bacteria, or environmental pollutants, though the precise cause remains unknown in many cases. Viruses play a important aetiological role, with rhinoviruses being implicated most often. How many exacerbations are caused by bacteria is uncertain, as pathogenic bacteria can often be grown from the sputum of clinically stable patients. However, one suggestion is that the isolation of a new strain may be associated with development of an exacerbation.

Management

Oxygen therapy
Patients admitted to hospital with an exacerbation should be given oxygen to maintain the saturation of arterial blood at >90%. For patients with type 2 respiratory failure, give controlled oxygen (24% or 28%) through a Venturi facemask. For patients with type 1 respiratory failure, titrate the oxygen concentration upwards to maintain a saturation of >90%. After giving oxygen for 30-60 minutes, recheck arterial blood gases, especially in those with type 2 respiratory failure. This allows detection of rising carbon dioxide concentration or falling pH due to loss of hypoxic drive.

Bronchodilators
Bronchodilators are a fundamental component in managing exacerbations, and all patients should be given inhaled salbutamol. Salbutamol stimulates β_2 adrenoceptors to cause smooth muscle relaxation and bronchodilation. Although there are few data to support any additional benefit in acute exacerbations, the short acting anticholinergic ipratropium may be given concomitantly. Both bronchodilators have a duration of action of between four and six hours and are generally well tolerated.

Differential diagnosis of an exacerbation of COPD

- Exacerbation of asthma
- Bronchopneumonia
- Pulmonary embolism
- Pleural effusion
- Bronchial carcinoma
- Bronchiectasis
- Pneumothorax
- Upper airway obstruction
- Pulmonary oedema
- Cardiac arrhythmia, such as atrial fibrillation

Investigations for patients admitted to hospital with exacerbation of COPD

- Full blood count
- Blood biochemistry and glucose concentration
- Theophylline plasma concentration (in patients using a theophylline preparation)
- Arterial blood gas (documenting the fraction of inspired oxygen)
- Electrocardiography
- Chest radiography
- Blood cultures in febrile patients
- Microscopy, culture and sensitivity of purulent sputum

Possible causes of an exacerbation of COPD

Bacteria	Viruses	Pollutants
• *Haemophilus influenzae*	• Rhinovirus	• Ozone
• *Streptococcus pneumoniae*	• Influenza	• Sulphur dioxide
• *Haemophilus parainfluenzae*	• Parainfluenza	• Nitrogen dioxide
• *Moraxella catarrhalis*	• Respiratory syncytial virus	
• *Pseudomonas aeruginosa*	• Coronavirus	

Arterial blood gas features of types 1 and 2 respiratory failure

	Respiratory failure	
	Type 1	**Type 2**
O_2	Lowered	Lowered
CO_2	Normal or lowered	Raised
HCO_3	Normal	Raised or normal
pH	Normal or raised	Normal or lowered

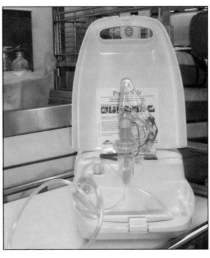

Nebulised bronchodilators are often given during an exacerbation of COPD

Bronchodilators can be administered successfully via a metered dose inhaler plus spacer or a nebuliser. Although a nebuliser does not confer any advantage in drug delivery over hand held devices with a spacer, it is independent of patient effort and often more convenient in a busy ward. In patients with hypercapnia or respiratory acidosis, nebulisers should usually be driven by compressed air and supplemental oxygen given via a nasal cannula.

Corticosteroids

Unless they are contraindicated, oral corticosteroids should be given to all patients with an exacerbation of COPD. Several studies have shown that they improve lung function and shorten the length of hospital stay. Severely ill patients or those who are unable to swallow can initially be given 100-200 mg of intravenous hydrocortisone. For straightforward exacerbations, current guidelines recommend that 30-40 mg of prednisolone is given for 7-14 days, with no additional benefit being gained with longer courses of treatment. Instruct patients on when and how to discontinue oral corticosteroids and be aware of potential adverse effects (discussed in article 7 of this series). Patients taking oral corticosteroids for less than three weeks do not usually need to taper off the dose.

Antibiotics

Despite viruses and pollutants being implicated in many exacerbations of COPD, antibiotics are still widely used. Antibiotics are most effective in severe exacerbations with increased sputum volume and purulence. It is important to tailor the choice of antibiotic to local patterns of sensitivity and resistance, although amoxicillin is a suitable first choice. Patients who are allergic to penicillin should be given a macrolide (such as erythromycin or clarithromycin).

Aminophylline

Aminophylline has only modest benefits at best in treating exacerbations of COPD, and its use is controversial. In a meta-analysis of four trials, aminophylline in conjunction with conventional treatment failed to confer any advantage over placebo in terms of lung function, symptoms, or length of hospital stay. However, its use was associated with a greater incidence of adverse effects such as nausea and vomiting.

Current guidelines suggest adding aminophylline to standard therapy for patients with moderate to severe exacerbations or those not responding to nebulised bronchodilators.

Respiratory stimulants

Since the introduction of non-invasive ventilation the use of doxapram has become far less common in hypercapnic respiratory failure. It may have some use if non-invasive ventilation is contraindicated or not immediately available, but whether it confers benefit when used alongside non-invasive ventilation is uncertain. Doxapram is given by continuous intravenous infusion and stimulates both respiratory and non-respiratory muscles. Its use is often limited by adverse effects such as agitation, tachycardia, confusion, and hallucinations.

Non-invasive ventilation

Non-invasive ventilation has revolutionised the management of hypercapnic respiratory failure due to COPD and will be discussed in the next article in this series.

General hospital care

Measures to prevent venous thromboembolism with low molecular weight heparin should be considered in all patents

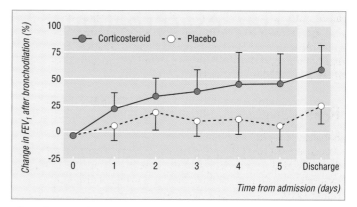

Effect of oral corticosteroids compared with placebo on forced expiratory volume in one second (FEV_1) of patients with an exacerbation of COPD

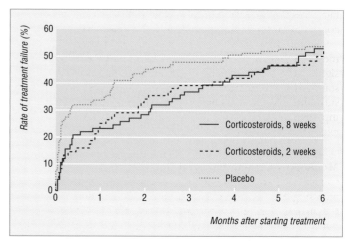

Effects of oral corticosteroids for an exacerbation of COPD, showing no difference between short and long courses (2 and 8 weeks) on rates of treatment failure

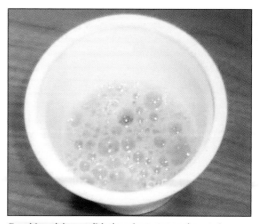

Consider giving antibiotics when sputum is purulent and of greater volume than usual

---

Guidance for adding aminophylline to standard therapy for COPD exacerbations

Patients not taking oral theophylline
- Give loading dose of 5 mg/kg over ≥ 20 minutes with cardiac monitoring
- Subsequent maintenance infusion of 0.5 mg/kg/hour

Patients already taking theophylline
- Omit loading dose of aminophylline
- Before starting maintenance infusion of 0.5 mg/kg/hour, plasma concentration of theophylline should ideally be obtained
- Measure daily plasma theophylline concentration and alter infusion rate to maintain a concentration of 10-20 mg/l (55-110 μmol/l).

admitted with an exacerbation of COPD. Attention should also be given to adequate hydration and nutritional input. Many patients with COPD have important comorbidities—such as ischaemic heart disease, left ventricular dysfunction, and diabetes—which must not be overlooked.

Recovery

Assisted hospital discharge

Any intervention that hastens a patient's recovery and discharge from hospital may be useful in the overall management of an exacerbation. In recent years, "assisted hospital discharge" schemes have been developed whereby patients with non-severe exacerbations of COPD can be discharged almost immediately with appropriate nursing and medical back up. As well as providing patients with a package of care, this practice also facilitates the identification of a deterioration in clinical condition and readmission to hospital if necessary.

Studies have shown that rates of hospital readmission and mortality among patients on assisted discharge schemes are not significantly different from those among individuals receiving standard inpatient care. Moreover, such schemes have produced substantial cost savings and increased the availability of inpatient beds. However, not all patients admitted with an exacerbation of COPD are suitable for assisted discharge.

Monitoring while in hospital

Clinical assessment and routine observations are useful in assessing the rate of recovery from an exacerbation. Frequent measuring of arterial blood gases is required to monitor patients with decompensated respiratory acidosis. Daily recordings of peak expiratory flow rates are less useful unless the patient has reversible obstructive lung disease. It is useful to record spirometry before discharge as this helps to confirm the diagnosis (in patients who have not previously had it performed), provides information on the severity of airflow obstruction, and allows progress to be assessed at subsequent outpatient follow-up.

Outpatient follow-up

Arrange hospital outpatient clinic follow up for four to six weeks after discharge in most patients. As well as allowing monitoring of changes in lung function, this is an opportunity to provide education, check inhaler technique, consider augmentation of pharmacotherapy, check oxygen saturation and arterial blood gases if required, and reassess smoking status.

Explain to patients that they should report symptoms suggestive of an exacerbation of COPD to their general practitioner at an early stage. This is important since early and prompt treatment results in a quicker recovery than if treatment is delayed. Moreover, patients who fail to recognise or promptly report worsening symptoms have a greater risk of being admitted to hospital and generally have a poorer quality of life.

Recurrent exacerbations

Many patients with COPD have frequent exacerbations, necessitating repeated hospital admissions. This is especially so for individuals with hypercapnic respiratory failure who have had treatment with non-invasive ventilation. Indeed, within a year after hospital discharge, most of these patients will be readmitted and require further non-invasive ventilation, with as many as half dying. Further studies are required to identify factors associated with readmission and to devise strategies to address this common problem.

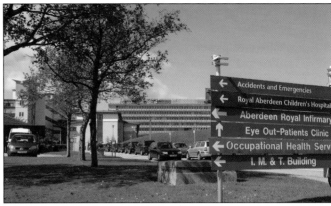

After discharge from hospital with an exacerbation of COPD, most patients should be reviewed at the hospital outpatient clinic

---

Relative contraindications to assisted hospital discharge in patients with an exacerbation of COPD

- Acute onset
- Confusion
- Worsening peripheral oedema
- Uncertain diagnosis
- Poor performance status
- Concomitant unstable medical disorders
- New chest radiograph abnormalities
- Acidosis or marked hypoxia or hypercapnia
- Adverse social conditions

Further reading

- McCrory DC, Brown CD. Anticholinergic bronchodilators versus beta2-sympathomimetic agents for acute exacerbations of chronic obstructive pulmonary disease. *Cochrane Database Syst Rev* 2002;(4): CD003900
- Wood-Baker RR, Gibson PG, Hannay M, Walters EH, Walters JAE. Systemic corticosteroids for acute exacerbations of chronic obstructive pulmonary disease. *Cochrane Database Syst Rev* 2005;(1) CD001288
- Duffy N, Walker P, Diamantea F, Calverley PMA, Davies L. Intravenous aminophylline in patients admitted to hospital with non-acidotic exacerbations of chronic obstructive pulmonary disease: a prospective randomised controlled trial. *Thorax* 2005;60: 713-7
- Chu CM, Chan VL, Lin AWN, Wong IWY, Leung WS, Lai CKW. Readmission rates and life-threatening events in COPD survivors treated with non-invasive ventilation for hypercapnic respiratory failure. *Thorax* 2004;59:1020-5
- Wilkinson TMA, Donaldson GC, Hurst JR, Seemungal TAR, Wedzicha JA. Early therapy improves outcomes of exacerbations of chronic obstructive pulmonary disease. *Am J Resp Crit Care Med* 2004;168:1298-303

Competing interests: GPC has received funding for attending international conferences and honorariums for giving talks from pharmaceutical companies GlaxoSmithKline, Pfizer, and AstraZeneca. JAW has received funding or honorariums for giving lectures or attending advisory boards from GlaxoSmithKline, AstraZeneca, Aventis Pasteur, Bayer, Boehringer Ingelheim, Novartis, Pfizer, and Arrow Therapeutics.

The figure of effects of oral corticosteroids on FEV₁ was adapted from Davies et al. *Lancet* 1999;354:456-60. The figure comparing short and long courses of oral corticosteroids was adapted from Niewoehner et al. *N Engl J Med* 1999;340:1941-7.

10 Ventilatory support

Gordon Christie, Graeme P Currie, Paul Plant

Non-invasive ventilation

The introduction and widespread use of non-invasive ventilation (NIV) has revolutionised the management and survival of patients with an acidotic exacerbation of chronic obstructive pulmonary disease (COPD). Indeed, it is difficult to justify admitting patients with an exacerbation of COPD to hospitals where NIV is not readily available. A close fitting facemask or nose mask connected to a portable ventilator facilitates a non-invasive method of providing respiratory support to a spontaneously breathing patient. The mask can be removed easily, allowing patients to communicate, eat, drink, and take nebulised and oral drugs.

How non-invasive ventilation works

NIV provides a two level form of respiratory support, supplying inspiratory and expiratory positive airways pressure.

Inspiratory positive airways pressure, which is usually titrated up to 15-20 cm H_2O, helps offload tiring respiratory muscles and reduce the work of breathing, improves alveolar ventilation and oxygenation, and increases elimination of CO_2.

Expiratory positive airways pressure, usually at 4-6 cm H_2O, helps "splint open" the airway and flushes CO_2 from the mask. It also reduces the work of breathing by overcoming intrinsic positive end expiratory pressure, thereby reducing atelectasis and increasing the end tidal volume.

Oxygen is introduced either through a port in the facemask or through a more proximal channel in the ventilator system. It is not usually necessary to deliver humidified oxygen, but humidifiers can be added to the circuit.

When to use non-invasive ventilation in COPD

NIV is particularly successful in patients with hypercapnic respiratory failure (especially in those with an arterial blood pH of 7.25-7.35). It can also be used as a therapeutic trial before proceeding to mechanical ventilation or when more invasive ventilatory support is inappropriate. In the latter circumstance, NIV is therefore considered the "ceiling of treatment."

Studies with various end points—such as mortality, need for intubation, arterial blood gases, and cost effectiveness—have consistently shown significant benefits with NIV. For example, a meta-analysis of eight randomised controlled trials evaluated effects of NIV in patients admitted with an exacerbation of COPD with an arterial CO_2 pressure (PaCO$_2$) of >6 kPa. Compared with standard treatment alone, concomitant NIV reduced mortality, need for intubation, likelihood of treatment failure, and complication rate. It also produced improvements in blood pH, PaCO$_2$, and respiratory rate within an hour and resulted in a shorter stay in hospital.

Setting

NIV can be used in hospital wards and in high dependency and intensive care units. It can be started in accident and emergency departments, but in many such cases, patients will not have had sufficient time to respond to conventional treatment. The exact setting is less important than the availability of experienced nurses, physiotherapists, and medical staff to start treatment, monitor progress, and troubleshoot. In the treatment of COPD, there is little to guide choice of ventilator other than familiarity,

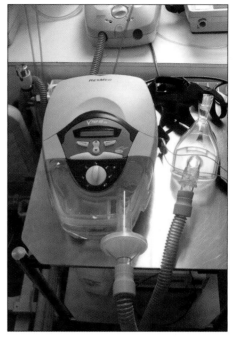

Non-invasive ventilation can be given using a full facemask or nose mask

---

Advantages of non-invasive ventilation over invasive mechanical ventilation

- Patients can eat and drink
- Patients can communicate and make decisions about management
- A physiological cough is maintained
- Physiological warming and humidification occurs
- No sedatives are required
- Reduced risk of ventilator associated pneumonia
- Less expensive, and intensive care bed not necessarily required
- Allows intermittent use, which facilitates weaning

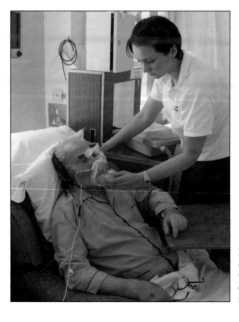

Non-invasive ventilation can be used in hospital wards and in high dependency and intensive care units

cost, and local preference. If NIV is used for hypoxic respiratory failure the ventilator unit needs an intrinsic blender to ensure delivery of high fractions of inspired oxygen. Intensive care ventilators are often difficult to use non-invasively as they are poorly tolerant of leaks and alarm readily.

How to use non-invasive ventilation

Before starting NIV, decide whether the patient is a suitable candidate for invasive mechanical ventilation and document the decision. Also discuss with the patient and his or her family whether they would wish further respiratory support if NIV proves unsuccessful.

Explain what you are about to do. Providing the clinical condition permits, show the patient the ventilator, facemask, and tubing. Choose an appropriately sized facemask (sizing rings are usually provided by the manufacturer). Nasal masks are more comfortable, but require patients to breathe through their nose. Most patients with acute exacerbations of COPD breathe through their mouth, and full facemasks are therefore preferable. It is useful if the mask is firstly placed on the patient's face for several minutes before securing it with straps.

Set the oxygen to an appropriate initial flow rate (typically 1-2 l/min) and titrate it upwards to maintain a saturation of at least 90%. Set both inspiratory and expiratory positive airways pressures, usually starting at 10 and 4 cm H_2O respectively. The inspiratory pressure can then be titrated up to 15-20 cm H_2O or to the maximum pressure comfortably tolerated by the patient. Depending on the type of ventilator, other parameters may be set, such as the sensitivity of the inspiratory and expiratory triggers and maximum inspiratory and expiratory times. These may need adjustment to maximise synchrony between the ventilator and the patient's efforts. Good synchrony makes for efficient ventilation and greater comfort for the patient. For some patients with shallow breathing or low respiratory rates, it may be necessary to programme the ventilator to deliver a minimum number of breaths per minute.

Monitoring non-invasive ventilation

Irrespective of PaO_2 or $PaCO_2$, the arterial blood pH is a reliable marker of severity in exacerbations of COPD and is closely linked to mortality and need for intubation. As well as regularly recording pulse, blood pressure, and respiratory rate, continuously monitor oxygen saturation.

Check arterial blood gases one hour after starting NIV; an improvement in blood pH or $PaCO_2$ and reduction in respiratory rate are good prognostic signs. If no improvement occurs, check that the patient is wearing the mask, that it is comfortable without excessive leak, and that the ventilator is in synchrony with the patient's respiratory effort, and then consider adjusting the ventilator settings (such as inspiratory pressure or oxygen flow rate). Blood gases should be rechecked within four hours of a change in setting, or earlier in the event of a clinical deterioration.

Weaning from NIV is rarely a problem, as patients normally "auto wean" by progressively decreasing their use after a few days.

Other measures

Institute maximal drug treatment—such as nebulised bronchodilators, corticosteroids, and antibiotics—in patients starting NIV. Check whether patients are using sedative drugs such as benzodiazepines and opiates: if so, these may require pharmacological reversal, especially if the respiratory rate is low. Keep patients adequately hydrated and maintain an adequate calorific intake.

Factors to consider in deciding a patient's suitability for invasive mechanical ventilation

- Presence of concomitant medical conditions
- Premorbid functional status
- Severity of existing airflow obstruction
- Presence of potentially reversible precipitant (such as pneumonia or pneumothorax)
- Patient and family wishes

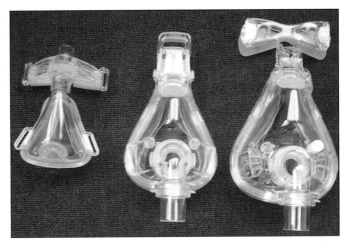

A variety of face masks sizes or, less commonly, nose masks are available for use with NIV

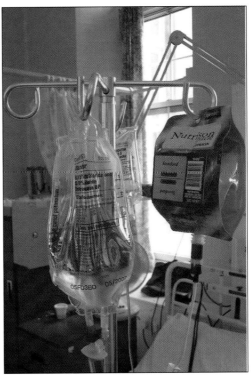

Patients receiving NIV can easily become dehydrated and undernourished; adequate hydration and nutrition should not be forgotten in the overall management

Before the introduction of NIV, doxapram was often used as a respiratory stimulant. Few studies have made direct comparisons with NIV, but doxapram has only limited ability to improve blood gas tensions. Moreover, a high incidence of adverse effects means that it is often poorly tolerated. Its role alongside NIV is not established, and it should not be used except under specialist supervision. However, it may be used as a temporising measure if NIV is not immediately available or cannot be tolerated.

Problems with non-invasive ventilation

Most patients tolerate NIV without serious problems, but some have difficulty "breathing with the machine." The facemask can cause problems such as claustrophobia, facial sores, and persistent air leaks. There are few absolute contraindications to NIV, and all patients' suitability should be assessed on an individual basis. With moribund patients, however, consider whether either intubation or a palliative approach might be more appropriate. Patients who recover from an exacerbation treated with NIV are at high risk of a future exacerbation and should be asked whether they would wish ventilatory support in the future.

Domiciliary non-invasive ventilation

The role of domiciliary NIV in COPD is controversial. Unlike patients with neuromuscular disorders, patients with COPD tend to be poorly compliant once at home. Randomised controlled trials have failed to show either a definite survival advantage or improvement in quality of life. However, for hypoxic patients with COPD who develop hypercapnia or acidosis while receiving long term oxygen therapy, domiciliary nocturnal NIV may be useful. It can also be useful for patients with hypercapnic respiratory failure who are frequently admitted to hospital with exacerbations associated with acidosis.

Mechanical ventilation

Invasive mechanical ventilation should be considered in patients whose pH, $PaCO_2$, and respiratory rate have deteriorated or failed to improve within four hours of initiation of NIV. NIV is less likely to be successful in such patients, or in those with severe acidosis such as an initial pH < 7.26. Moreover, patients who remain acidotic 48 hours after starting treatment with NIV tend to have a poor prognosis. Such patients have a higher mortality if NIV is continued than if mechanical ventilation is initiated, and the latter treatment should therefore be considered.

Long term survival in patients with COPD who require mechanical ventilation is generally lower than in those who require NIV alone. However, failure of NIV should not be used as a reason to decline invasive mechanical ventilation and does not imply that these patients will be difficult to wean. For patients who cannot be weaned on to NIV within 48-72 hours of starting mechanical ventilation, early fashioning of a tracheostomy may facilitate weaning and reduce the time spent in intensive care.

Competing interests: GPC has received funding for attending international conferences and honorariums for giving talks from pharmaceutical companies GlaxoSmithKline, Pfizer, and AstraZeneca.

Relative contraindications to using non-invasive ventilation

- Orofacial burns
- Recent orofacial surgery
- Bowel obstruction
- Decreased consciousness
- Copious respiratory secretions
- Cardiovascular instability
- Untreated pneumothorax
- Agitation
- Persistent vomiting
- Unstable upper airway
- Severe respiratory acidosis

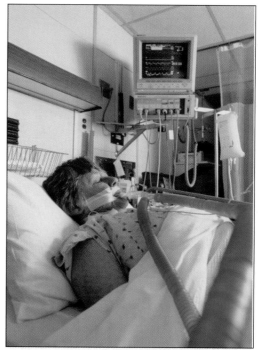

Deciding when to abandon NIV and start invasive mechanical ventilation is often difficult

---

Further reading
- Non-invasive ventilation in acute respiratory failure. *Thorax* 2002; 57:192-211
- Plant PK, Owen JL, Elliott MW. Early use of non-invasive ventilation for acute exacerbations of chronic obstructive pulmonary disease on general respiratory wards: a multicentre randomised controlled trial. *Lancet* 2000;355:1931-5
- Lightowler JV, Wedzicha JA, Elliott MW, Ram FS. Non-invasive positive pressure ventilation to treat respiratory failure resulting from exacerbations of chronic obstructive pulmonary disease: Cochrane systematic review and meta-analysis. *BMJ* 2003;326:185

The figure of invasive mechanical ventilation is supplied by Custom Medical Stock and the Science Photo Library.

11 Primary care and palliative care

Daryl Freeman, David Price

Primary care

Over the past decade, interest in diagnosing and managing COPD in primary care has grown in recognition of its increasing burden on patients, families, health services, and society. Guidelines from bodies such as the British Thoracic Society, National Institute for Health and Clinical Excellence, Global Initiative for Chronic Obstructive Lung Disease, and International Primary Care Airways Group have also increased awareness of COPD among primary care doctors.

COPD is a cause of great misery to many patients and their carers. Decreasing lung function—with symptoms such as breathlessness, cough, wheeze, fluid retention, and fatigue—results in a downward spiral of reduced activity, social isolation, loss of independence, depression, and increased contact with health and social care providers. However, considerable help can and should be provided in primary care. Recently, the inclusion of COPD management in the UK general practice "new contract" has provided incentives for better care.

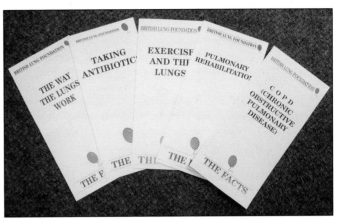

All patients should receive education about COPD

Detection

Patients with COPD typically present late, often with respiratory tract infections that have not previously been linked with COPD or with breathlessness misdiagnosed as asthma. Studies suggest that, among cigarette smokers older than 40 years, about 20% of those without a respiratory diagnosis and at least a quarter of those with a diagnosis of asthma actually have COPD. By the time most have COPD diagnosed, at least 50% of their lung function will have been lost.

Thus, a priority in primary care should be earlier detection and correct diagnosis. The use of simple questionnaires may allow easier detection of patients who need spirometry, avoiding the need for mass spirometry screening programmes.

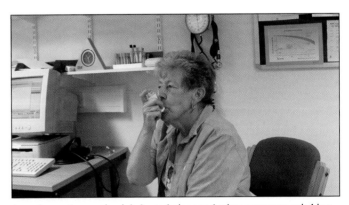

Assessing and correcting inhaler technique and, when necessary, switching to an alternative device are vital in all patients with COPD

Simple questionnaire for evaluating risk of COPD

Patient characteristic	Value	Score*
Age (years)?	40-49	0
	50-59	4
	60-69	8
	≥70	10
Smoking pack years?	0-14	0
	15-24	2
	25-49	3
	≥50	7
Body mass index?	<25.4	5
	25.4-29.7	1
	>29.7	0
Cough affected by weather?	Yes	3
	No or no cough	0
Sputum production in absence of a cold?	Yes	3
	No	0
Sputum production first thing in the morning?	Yes	0
	No	3
Wheezes?	Sometimes or often	4
	Never	0
Has or used to have any allergies?	Yes	0
	No	3

*Total scores of ≥17 suggest increased risk of COPD being present

Simple questionnaire for differential diagnosis of COPD

Patient characteristic	Value	Score*
Age (years)?	40-49	0
	50-59	5
	60-69	9
	≥70	11
Smoking pack years?	0-14	0
	15-24	3
	25-49	7
	≥50	9
Increased frequency of cough in recent years?	Yes	0
	No	1
Breathing problems in past 3 years?†	Yes	0
	No	3
Ever admitted to hospital with breathing problems?	Yes	6
	No	0
Short of breath more often in recent years?	Yes	1
	No	0
How much sputum coughed up most days?	<15 ml/day	0
	≥15 ml/day	4
When gets a cold it usually goes to chest?	Yes	4
	No	0
Taking any treatment to help breathing?	Yes	5
	No	0

*Total scores of ≤18 suggest asthma is the predominant diagnosis, scores of ≥19 suggest COPD
†Serious enough to keep patient away from work, indoors, at home, or in bed

ABC of chronic obstructive pulmonary disease

Diagnosis and assessment

The diagnosis of COPD is established by detection of airflow obstruction in conjunction with typical symptoms and a history of smoking. Spirometry must be performed by adequately trained staff using a vitalograph that is properly maintained and calibrated. Similarly, results should be interpreted by individuals with sufficient expertise. Some primary care teams may find either performing or interpreting spirometry difficult, and help should be readily available in undertaking these tasks.

The severity of COPD should be assessed not only in terms of impairment in lung function but as an overall assessment of the patient. This should include symptoms (particularly breathlessness according to the MRC dyspnoea score), frequency of exacerbations, extent of disability, health status, evidence of depression and anxiety, and body mass index.

Secondary care referral

The decision to refer to secondary care will depend on the individual general practitioner's experience and confidence in managing COPD and on the facilities available. If diagnostic uncertainty exists, however, consider referral to a specialist to help confirm or refute the diagnosis. Other potential reasons for specialist referral include
- Severe airflow obstruction
- Marked functional impairment
- Rapidly declining lung function
- Assessment of suitability of domiciliary oxygen in hypoxic patients
- Young age or family history of α_1 antitrypsin deficiency
- Persistent symptoms despite apparently adequate therapy
- Frequent exacerbations and infections
- Haemoptysis or suspected lung cancer
- Signs suggestive of cor pulmonale
- Assessment for specialist treatment such as nebulisers, pulmonary rehabilitation, domiciliary non-invasive ventilation, lung volume reduction surgery, lung transplantation, or bullectomy.

Management of stable disease

Once the diagnosis of COPD has been established, ensure that patients are given sufficient information about the disorder and that their inhaler technique is assessed at every available opportunity. The detailed management of patients with stable COPD should involve both non-pharmacological and pharmacological measures as outlined in earlier articles. Pulmonary rehabilitation is not universally available, although in some regions it is extending beyond secondary care to community settings. This development may be especially attractive to patients with milder disease and those in rural communities where travelling to a secondary care centre every week for several months is impractical.

Management of exacerbations

Most exacerbations can and should be managed by the patient or the primary care team. The decision to admit a patient to hospital depends on a combination of physical and social criteria, which may vary according to the facilities available to the clinician making the decision. Patients may find a self management plan useful. This normally gives advice on how to recognise and respond to an exacerbation. Its content will probably vary according to the patient population (and indeed individual patients) but should include
- How to recognise an exacerbation
- What treatment to take and for how long (antibiotics, oral corticosteroids, and increase in bronchodilators)

MRC dyspnoea score	
Grade	**Impact of dyspnoea**
1	Not troubled by breathlessness except on vigorous exertion
2	Short of breath when hurrying or walking up inclines
3	Walks slower than contemporaries because of breathlessness, or has to stop for breath when walking at own pace
4	Stops for breath after walking about 100 metres or stops after a few minutes' walking on the level
5	Too breathless to leave the house or breathless on dressing or undressing

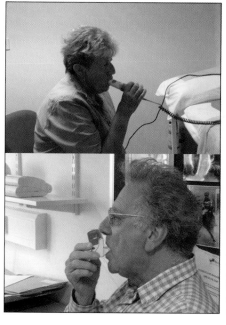

A patient's lung function can be assessed in primary care with a benchtop vitalograph (top) or a handheld device (bottom)

Suggested format for initial assessment of a patient with COPD

Diagnosis and severity
- Date diagnosis confirmed
- Spirometry
- Severity
- Body mass index
- MRC dyspnoea score

Medical history
- Respiratory
- Cardiac
- Other

Smoking status
- Date stopped
- Smoking pack years
- Smoking cessation advice

Investigations
- Full blood count
- Chest radiograph
- Oxygen saturation (%)

Exacerbations in past 12 months
- No of antibiotic courses
- No of oral corticosteroid courses
- No of hospital admissions

Treatment review
- Patient's understanding of treatment
- Inhaler technique
- Self management plan
- Oxygen therapy

Vaccinations
- Influenza
- Pneumococcal

Holistic review
- Depression
- Vulnerable patient (lives alone or severe disease)

Referral to other teams or services
- Secondary care
- Community nursing teams
- Palliative care services
- Osteoporosis assessment

Time to next review

- Who to contact in an emergency (including out of hours services, or the nearest emergency room facility) and how to recognise the need to do so
- Advice to see their doctor or respiratory nurse for review once they have improved.

Structured review

The need to review patients with COPD will depend on the individual patient, the severity and stability of the disease, the extent of social support, and any recent changes in treatment. However, all patients should be reviewed four to six weeks after a change in treatment or after an exacerbation (this should include measurement of spirometry, a review of treatment, and discussion of patients' understanding of their disease). In general, those with mild to moderate disease should be reviewed annually, while those with severe disease at least every six months. The review process may be assisted by the use of standardised templates for primary care computer systems such as that endorsed by the General Practice Airways Group (www.gpiag.org/news/copd_template1.php).

Palliative care

Palliative care can be defined as "an approach that improves quality of life of patients and their families facing the problems associated with life threatening illness, through the prevention and relief of suffering by means of early identification and impeccable assessment and treatment of pain and other problems, physical, psychosocial and spiritual."

Patients with end stage COPD need structured palliative care at least as much as patients with malignant disease, and this should ideally be delivered by a multidisciplinary team working in synchrony. In some cases referral to a specialist palliative care team with access to hospice beds and home nursing services may be required. However, primary care input is vital as the individual patient's general practice will probably have looked after the patient for many years and be familiar with his or her family and social background. Knowing when to discuss prognosis is often difficult, as patients vary widely in the length of time between diagnosis and pre-terminal events. However, most patients generally find open discussion about end of life issues worth while and prefer to be involved in decision making.

Symptom control

The most disturbing symptom for patients with end stage COPD is usually overwhelming dyspnoea, which often induces anxiety and frank fear. General principles for management of distressing breathlessness revolve around reassuring patients and care givers, suggesting distraction techniques, devising coping strategies, adapting daily activities, and ensuring patients have realistic expectations of their capabilities. Some patients find that a moving stream of cool air produced by a bedside or hand held fan also helps to relieve breathlessness, but oxygen should be considered if patients are hypoxic. Patients should, of course, receive bronchodilators. For individuals with end stage disease who continue to have distressing breathlessness despite maximal treatment, there should be a low threshold to starting opiates and benzodiazepines. However, palliation of symptoms should neither postpone nor hasten death.

Patients at the pre-terminal stage who are too weak to expectorate may experience accumulations of upper airway secretions. These can produce a "death rattle" that may be distressing to both patient and family. In hospital, oropharyngeal suctioning may be useful, and if this fails a subcutaneous infusion or boluses of hyoscine hydrobromide can be given (0.6-2.4 mg/24 hours).

Suggested format for structured review of a patient with COPD

Smoking status
- Is patient still smoking?
  If no: date stopped and pack year exposure
  If yes: smoking cessation advice offered and response and current pack year exposure

Treatment review
- Patient's understanding of treatment
- Inhaler technique
- Self management plan discussed and reviewed
- Oxygen therapy

Assess impairment and severity
- Repeat spirometry
- Oxygen saturation (%)
- Body mass index

Assess symptoms
- MRC dyspnoea score

Exacerbations in past 12 months
- No of antibiotic courses
- No of oral corticosteroid courses
- No of hospital admissions

Holistic review
- Depression or anxiety
- Social situation

Assess need to refer to other teams or services
- Secondary care
- Community nursing teams
- Palliative care
- Osteoporosis assessment

Time to next review
- Change in treatment: 6 weeks
- No change in treatment: 3-9 months depending on severity

Drugs for symptom control in end stage COPD

Opiates and benzodiazepines are the most useful drugs in relieving breathlessness in end stage disease

Opiates
- Useful in reducing the sensation of breathlessness
- Initially prescribe oral morphine (for example, Oramorph or Sevredol 2.5-5 mg) as required
- This can lead on to a regular longer acting opiate

Benzodiazepines
- Useful in relieving breathlessness when anxiety is an integral component
- Can be prescribed alone or alongside opiates
- Lorazepam can be used sublingually as required at dose of 0.5-1 mg
- Patients with persistent anxiety or breathlessness may require a regular longer acting benzodiazepine such as diazepam 2-5 mg every 8 hours

---

Further reading

- Bellamy D, Bouchard J, Henrichsen S, Johansson G, Langhammer A, Reid J, et al. International Primary Care Respiratory Group (IPCRG) guidelines: management of chronic obstructive pulmonary disease (COPD). *Prim Care Respir J* 2006;15:48-57
- Abernethy AP, Currow DC, Frith P, Fazekas BS, McHugh A, Bui C. Randomised, double blind, placebo controlled crossover trial of sustained release morphine for the management of refractory dyspnoea. *BMJ* 2003;327:523-8
- Davies CL. ABC of palliative care: Breathlessness, cough, and other respiratory symptoms. *BMJ* 1997;315:931-4

Competing interests: DF has received travel grants to national and international conferences, reimbursement for lecturing and speaking at educational meetings, and funding for clinical staff from GlaxoSmithKline, Boehringer Ingelheim, Schering Plough, Altana, and AstraZeneca. DP has received honorariums for speaking at sponsored meetings or attending advisory boards and research funding from 3M, Altana, AstraZeneca, Boehringer Ingelheim, GlaxoSmithKline, Merck Sharp & Dohme, Novartis, Pfizer, Schering Plough, and Viatris. GPC has received funding for attending international conferences and honorariums for giving talks from pharmaceutical companies GlaxoSmithKline, Pfizer, and AstraZeneca.

The questionnaires for evaluating risk and differential diagnosis of COPD were adapted from Price et al. *Chest* 2006;129:1531-9.

12 Future treatments

Peter J Barnes

Current treatment used in the management of chronic obstructive pulmonary disease (COPD) is often poorly effective and fails to halt the relentless decline in lung function that leads to increasing symptoms, disability, and exacerbations. This has stimulated clinicians, scientists, and drug companies to seek more effective ways to control the underlying disease process.

The challenge of drug development

Only recently has there been much research into the molecular and cell biology of COPD in order to identify new therapeutic targets. There are several reasons why drug development in COPD is fraught with difficulty, but significant progress is being been made, and several new therapeutic strategies are now in the preclinical and clinical stages of development.

New bronchodilators

The mainstay of current drug therapy in COPD consists of long acting bronchodilators—β_2 agonists (salmeterol and formoterol) and anticholinergics (tiotropium). These drugs are the preferred first line treatment for symptomatic patients with established disease. Several new long acting anticholinergics and once daily ("ultra-long acting") β_2 agonists are in development for treating COPD. Although novel classes of bronchodilators, such as potassium channel openers, have been investigated, these have proved to be less effective than established bronchodilators and have more adverse effects.

Fixed combination inhalers—which contain an inhaled corticosteroid plus long acting β_2 agonist—are now commonly prescribed for patients with COPD. Both salmeterol-fluticasone (Seretide) and formoterol-budesonide (Symbicort) are more effective than their separate constituents as monotherapy and are indicated in patients with moderate to severe airflow obstruction (forced expiratory volume in one second (FEV$_1$) <50% predicted) who have frequent exacerbations (>2 per year). Fixed combination inhalers containing a long acting corticosteroid and long acting β_2 agonist, which may be suitable for once daily treatment, are now in development.

When used on a once daily basis, the addition of formoterol to tiotropium has an additive effect on lung function. This is likely to pave the way for a fixed combination inhaler containing both a long acting anticholinergic plus long acting β_2 agonist.

Effective smoking cessation strategies

Cigarette smoking is the main cause of COPD, and quitting at most stages of the disease reduces progression. Smoking cessation is therefore an important part of management, although current cessation strategies have only limited long term success. One of the most effective drug treatments currently available is bupropion. However, in patients with COPD, an annual quit rate of around 15% indicates that more effective smoking cessation therapies are urgently required.

Several new classes of non-nicotinic drugs for smoking cessation are now in development. Some of these are based on altering neurotransmitter systems in the brain stem that are

---

Problems encountered in developing new drugs for treating COPD

- Animal models of COPD for early drug testing are unsatisfactory
- Methodological uncertainties exist about how best to test drugs for COPD in clinical trials, since long term studies (more than three years) with large numbers of patients may be required
- Many individuals with COPD have important comorbidities—such as ischaemic heart disease, left ventricular dysfunction, and diabetes—which might exclude them from clinical trials and therefore create doubts about the relevance of the trial results for "real life" patients
- There is little information about surrogate biomarkers—such as markers in blood, sputum, or breath—that could monitor the short term efficacy and predict the long term potential of new treatments

---

Current and future long acting bronchodilators for treating COPD

Long acting β_2 agonists
- Salmeterol (twice daily)*
- Formoterol (once daily)*
- TA 2005 (once daily)
- Indacaterol (once daily)
- GSK-159797 (once daily)

Long acting anticholinergics
- Tiotropium (once daily)*
- Glycopyrrolate (once daily)
- LAS34273 (once daily)

Combination inhalers
- Salmeterol-fluticasone (Seretide)*
- Formoterol-budesonide (Symbicort)*
- Formoterol-tiotropium

*Already marketed for treating COPD

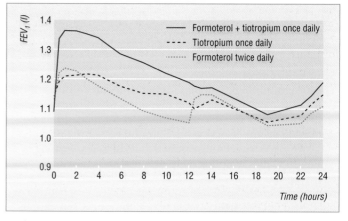

Additive effects of once daily formoterol and tiotropium on forced expiratory volume in 1 second (FEV$_1$) in patients with severe COPD after six weeks' treatment

---

Current and future drug treatments for smoking cessation

Current therapies
- Nicotine replacement therapy
- Bupropion

Future therapies
- Cannabinoid CB$_1$-receptor antagonists (such as rimonabant)
- Partial nicotine agonist (such as varenicline)
- GABA$_B$ antagonists
- Dopamine D$_3$ antagonists
- Nicotine vaccination (such as nic-Vax)

involved in "reward," but the prospects for long term efficacy seem limited as their action stops on withdrawal of treatment in animal models. However, rimonabant, a cannabinoid CB₁ antagonist currently in phase III trials, and varenicline, a partial nicotine agonist that targets the $\alpha_4\beta_2$ nicotinic acetylcholine receptor, seem to be promising in clinical trials.

An approach that may have longer term benefits is the development of a vaccine against nicotine. This stimulates the production of antibodies that bind nicotine, preventing it from entering the brain.

Treating inflammation in COPD

COPD is characterised by chronic inflammation, particularly of the small airways and lung parenchyma. With a predominance of macrophages, neutrophils, and cytotoxic T lymphocytes and inflammatory mediators, this inflammation has a different pattern from that of asthma, and, in sharp contrast, it is largely resistant to the anti-inflammatory effects of corticosteroids, prompting the search for alternative treatments. Better understanding of the underlying mechanisms in COPD has revealed several potential targets for non-steroidal anti-inflammatory agents.

Mediator antagonists
Many mediators—including lipid mediators and cytokines—are implicated in the pathophysiology of COPD. Inhibiting specific mediators, by receptor antagonists or synthesis inhibitors, is relatively easy, but such an approach is unlikely to produce effective drugs, since so many mediators with similar effects are involved. As a result of specific mediators having been shown to be increased in COPD, several mediator antagonists are in clinical development. Antibodies to tumour necrosis factor are used to treat severe rheumatoid arthritis and inflammatory bowel disease, but their effect on COPD is disappointing. An antibody that blocks interleukin 8 also seems to be largely ineffective.

Oxidative stress is increased in COPD, particularly as the disease becomes more advanced and during exacerbations. Oxidative stress amplifies inflammation and may result in corticosteroid resistance, and is therefore an important target for future treatment. Currently available antioxidants are not effective, and more potent and stable antioxidants—such as analogues of superoxide dismutase—are now in development.

Protease inhibitors
Several proteases—such as elastases, which are implicated in alveolar destruction—might be targeted to treat patients with COPD who have marked emphysema. Proteases may be inhibited by giving the endogenous antiprotease, such as α₁ antitrypsin, or by small molecule inhibitors. However, no clinical studies have yet shown these approaches to have any effect.

New anti-inflammatory treatments
The most promising new anti-inflammatory agents for use in COPD are phosphodiesterase 4 (PDE4) inhibitors. These orally active drugs increase cyclic AMP concentrations in inflammatory cells and exhibit a broad spectrum of anti-inflammatory effects.

Although effective in animal models of COPD, PDE4 inhibitors (such as cilomilast and roflumilast) have so far proved disappointing in clinical trials. This is because the dose is limited by adverse effects—particularly nausea and gastrointestinal problems. However, in a large randomised, placebo controlled study of patients with COPD with a mean

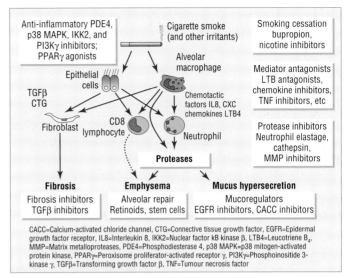

Inflammatory process in COPD. Inhaled irritants stimulate macrophages in the respiratory tract to release neutrophil chemotactic factors such as interleukin 8 and leucotriene B₄. These cells release proteases that break down connective tissue in lung parenchyma, leading to emphysema, and stimulate mucus hypersecretion. Cytotoxic (CD8) T cells may also be involved in alveolar wall destruction. White boxes show potential agents to inhibit stages in this process

Mediator antagonists for potential use in COPD

Mediator (role in COPD)	Inhibitor
Leucotriene B₄ (neutrophil chemotaxis)	Antagonists of leucotriene receptor BLT1 (such as BIIL284)
Interleukin 8 (neutrophil chemotaxis)	Blocking antibodies (such as ABX-IL8) Antagonists of interleukin receptor CXCR2 (such as GSK-656933)
Tumour necrosis factor α (amplifying inflammation)	Blocking antibodies (such as infliximab) Soluble receptors (such as etanercept)
Epidermal growth factor (mucus hypersecretion)	Receptor kinase inhibitors (such as gefitinib)
Oxidative stress (amplifying inflammation, resistance to corticosteroids)	Antioxidants (such as superoxide dismutase analogues)
Nitrative stress (resistance to corticosteroids)	Inducible nitric oxide synthase inhibitors (such as GSK-274150)

Protease inhibitors for potential use in COPD

Protease	Endogenous antiprotease	Small molecule inhibitor
Neutrophil elastase	α₁ antitrypsin	
	Secretory leucoprotease inhibitor	ONO-5046
	Elafin	
Cathepsins	Cystatins	Cysteine protease inhibitor
Matrix metalloproteases MMP-9	Tissue inhibitors of MMPs TIMP-1	Marimastat MMP-9 selective inhibitor

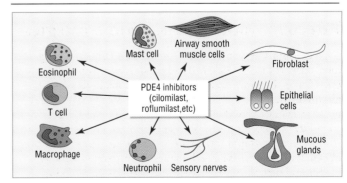

Broad spectrum of inhibitory effects of phosphodiesterase 4 (PDE4) inhibitors on inflammatory and structural cells in airways of patients with COPD

FEV$_1$ of around 50%, treatment with roflumilast reduced exacerbations and improved lung function over a 24 week period. Diarrhoea was the most common adverse effect largely due to active treatment and occurred in roughly 5% of patients. More selective inhibitors (PDE4B inhibitors) or inhaled administration of drugs are being investigated as ways to circumvent the problem of adverse effects.

Several other broad spectrum anti-inflammatory agents are currently under investigation, although most of these are likely to be associated with adverse effects when given systemically, suggesting that inhaled administration may be required.

Corticosteroid resistance is one of the typical features of COPD. An alternative therapeutic strategy is therefore to reverse the molecular mechanism of this resistance, which seems to be due to a defect in the nuclear enzyme histone deacetylase 2 (HDAC-2). This can be achieved in vitro with theophylline, which is an HDAC activator, or by inhibiting oxidative or nitrative stress. As a consequence, novel HDAC2 activators are now being sought.

Lung repair

COPD is a largely irreversible disease process, but it is possible that enhanced repair of damage might restore lung function in the future. There has been particular interest in retinoic acid, which is able to reverse experimental emphysema in rats. However, this is unlikely to work in humans, whose lungs do not have the regenerative capacity of that found in rats. Another approach now actively being explored is the use of stem cells in an attempt to regenerate alveolar type 1 cells.

Route of delivery

Drugs for airway diseases are traditionally given by inhalation, although inhaler devices usually target larger airways that are predominantly involved in asthma. Moreover, many elderly patients or those with musculoskeletal problems may have difficulty in using conventional inhalers. With COPD, the inflammation occurs mainly in the small airways and lung parenchyma, suggesting that devices that deliver drugs more peripherally may be of greater benefit. A systemic approach facilitated by oral drug delivery is therefore an attractive option. Oral treatments could also have an impact on systemic complications that are a problem in patients with severe disease, but this obviously carries an increased risk of adverse effects. An alternative approach is targeted drug delivery by exploiting specific cell uptake mechanisms in target cells, such as macrophages.

Novel anti-inflammatory treatments for COPD

- Phosphodiesterase 4 inhibitors (such as cilomilast, roflumilast)
- p38 mitogen-activated protein kinase inhibitors (such as SCIO-469)
- Nuclear factor κB inhibitors (such as AS602868)
- Phosphoinositide 3-kinase γ inhibitors
- Peroxisome proliferator-activated receptor γ agonists (such as rosiglitazone)
- Adhesion molecule inhibitors (such as bimosiamose)
- Non-antibiotic macrolides
- Resveratrol analogues

Reversal of corticosteroid resistance in COPD

- Theophylline (histone deacetylase activator)
- Histone deacetylase 2 selective activators
- Antioxidants
- Inducible nitric oxide synthase inhibitors
- Peroxynitrite scavengers

Further reading

- Barnes PJ, Hansel TT. Prospects for new drugs for chronic obstructive pulmonary disease. *Lancet* 2004;364:985-96
- Barnes PJ, Stockley RA. COPD: current therapeutic interventions and future approaches. *Eur Respir J* 2005;25:1084-106
- Rabe KF, Bateman ED, O'Donnell D, Witte S, Bredenbroker D, Bethke TD. Roflumilast—an oral anti-inflammatory treatment for chronic obstructive pulmonary disease: a randomised controlled trial. *Lancet* 2005;366:563-71

Competing interests: PJB has received research funding, speaker's fees, and consulting fees from several drug companies involved in developing new drugs for COPD, including GlaxoSmithKline, AstraZeneca, Boehringer Ingelheim, Novartis, Pfizer, Mitsubishi, Millennium, and Scios. GPC has received funding for attending international conferences and honorariums for giving talks from GlaxoSmithKline, Pfizer, and AstraZeneca.

The figure showing the additive effects of formoterol and tiotropium is adapted from van Noord JA, et al. *Eur Respir J* 2005;26:214-22. The figure of the inflammatory mechanisms in COPD and potential inhibitors and the figure of the effects of phosphodiesterase 4 inhibitors are adapted from Barnes PJ, Stockley RA. *Eur Respir J* 2005;25:1084-106.

Index

Index